"The [authors] consider such controversial matters as the safety of pesticides, children's needs for vitamin supplements and fiber, and the impact of television on obesity; concisely provide information about growth, nutrition, and fitness; and address such food-related issues as mealtime battles, junk-food consumption, food tensions during developmental stages, obesity, eating disorders, and food allergies. Their warm, no-nonsense presentation, based firmly on the scientific literature, even includes a chapter advising parents on interpreting media statements about food, diet, and nutrition."

—*Booklist*

"Combine[s] both good science and good sense."

—*Morning Sun*

"A refreshing look at kids and food."

—*Newsday*

What Should I Feed My Kids?

❖   ❖   ❖   ❖   ❖   ❖   ❖

The Pediatrician's Guide to Safe and
Healthy Food and Growth

(Formerly entitled *Let Them Eat Cake!*)

Ronald E. Kleinman, M.D.

Michael S. Jellinek, M.D.

WITH JULIE HOUSTON

FAWCETT COLUMBINE   •   NEW YORK

A Fawcett Columbine Book
Published by Ballantine Books

Copyright © 1994 by Julie Houston, Dr. Ronald Kleinman, and Dr. Michael Jellinek

*Grateful acknowledgment is made to the following for permission to reprint previously pub-
lished material:*
THE AMERICAN DIETETIC ASSOCIATION: Charts and text from *The Children's Food Safety Kit:
A Health Professional's Guide to the Issues*. Reprinted by permission of The National Center
for Nutrition and Dietetics of the American Dietetic Association.
CASTLEMEAD PUBLICATIONS: Height Velocity Chart for Boys (ref. #211) and Height Velocity
Chart for Girls (ref. #212), first published in the *Journal of Pediatrics*, vol. 107, 1985.
Copyright © 1985 by Castlemead Publications. Reprinted by permission.
THE NEW ENGLAND JOURNAL OF MEDICINE: Adaptation of an excerpt from David B. Herzog,
M.D., and Paul M. Copeland, M.D., "Eating Disorders" and chart "Criteria for Diagnosing
Anorexia Nervosa and Bulimia" from the same article [*The New England Journal of Medi-
cine*, vol. 313 (August 1, 1985), pp. 300–301]. Adapted and used by permission of David
Herzog, M.D., and *The New England Journal of Medicine*.
ROSS LABORATORIES: Eight NCHS growth charts adapted from P. V. V. Hamill, T. A. Drizd,
C. L. Johnson, R. B. Reed, A. F. Roche, and W. M. Moore, "Physical Growth: National
Center for Health Statistics Percentiles," *American Journal of Clinical Nutrition*, vol. 32
(1979), pages 607–29. Data from the National Center for Health Statistics (NCHS), Hy-
attsville, Maryland. Copyright © 1982 by Ross Laboratories. Reprinted by permission of
Ross Laboratories, Columbus, Ohio 43216.

Library of Congress Catalog Card Number: 95-90731

ISBN:0-449-90709-0

Cover design by Michelle T. Gengaro
Cover photograph © FPG International

Manufactured in the United States of America
First Ballantine Books Edition: March 1996
10 9 8 7 6 5 4 3 2 1

TO OUR FAMILIES:

MARTHA, ADAM, AND EMILY—R. E. K.

BARBARA, DAVID, ABRAHAM, ISAIAH, AND HANNAH ROSE—M. J.

CHARLIE, MOLLY, AND JAMES—J. H.

WITH DEEPEST AFFECTION

♦   ♦   ♦   ♦

Acknowledgments

We would like to acknowledge the wisdom and guidance of Dr. Laurence Finberg, whose dedication to the well-being of children and his contributions to our understanding of their nutritional needs has been invaluable.

To Dr. Terry Stoker, whose help in translating nutritional guidelines into sensible and reasonable recommendations can be seen throughout this book.

The section on eating disorders was largely drawn from Dr. David Herzog's extensive clinical work and publications.

Thanks to Beth Goldin, M.S.P.E., family fitness consultant and director of elementary physical education at the Berkeley Carroll School in Brooklyn, New York, for her input and editorial advice in shaping Chapter 10.

Finally, we wish to acknowledge the essential contributions of Ms. Helen Kiddy and Ms. Ellen Bean, whose dedication and helpful criticisms and support have made this manuscript possible.

Contents

What Should I Feed My Kids?

❖   ❖   ❖   ❖

Introduction

Children Caught in the Middle

Over the last few years, we have observed the curious phenom-
enon of children mimicking grown-ups as they debate various
food issues—discussing among themselves what is safe to eat
and what is harmful; what foods "have cholesterol," will "make
them fat" or "hyper" or "give them allergies." Clearly, these
children have been told by adults to follow certain rules about
food and diet—rules that often reflect adult confusion or
anxiety about their own food and health, rules frequently
based on misinformation and myth. As a result, many children
become caught in the middle of a no-win situation between
what they are told is right, i.e., to avoid "bad" foods and eat
certain others, and what they desire, to exercise choice and
explore new tastes. Either way, whether they have the foods
that are deemed "unhealthy" and thus disappoint their parents, or do not have them and feel deprived, their fun is
spoiled.

To put children in conflict over food choices creates unnecessary problems. Children are not middle-aged people and food is not a life-and-death issue for them. From a medical standpoint, if a child is growing normally, that child can enjoy a full, varied diet with little concern.

More important, no child should be made to feel guilty for what he or she eats. For whatever reasons, if a parent feels compelled to set rigid standards about food for him- or herself, the child is surely picking up on it. The parent's stress becomes the child's stress; the adult's guilt, the child's guilt. Children—even children who are not in the best of shape or who have health concerns—should not be made to feel bad about having pizza with friends before a movie, cotton candy at the circus, a burger with fries after soccer practice. Birthday parties should be special celebrations with friends—not just the rare chance to get chocolate cake, ice cream, and a party bag with candy in it.

Ironically, parents who are intensely committed to doing what is right for their children are often the ones who put their children under the most stress. Insisting on the "right" foods, the "right" schools and colleges, the "right" sports and after-school programs, families with very high standards can cause food restriction to become part of a pattern of overcontrol that is potentially quite destructive.

An extreme example of the effects of this type of overcontrol involves an eight-year-old girl who took showers two or three times a day and who told her parents she was so depressed she wanted to kill herself. This young girl was required to drink three glasses of milk a day to meet calcium needs, was never allowed Froot Loops or any other food with sugar, and for dessert usually had cut-up pieces of fruit. She had to buy candy bars and treats with her own money—but she didn't get an allowance. This child went to a very strict, highly competitive school that recommended their students be in bed no later than seven-thirty every night. Three times a week after school, she went to religious instruction. For relaxation at home, she played with educational toys—in her house, there was no television, Nintendo, or Macintosh games to blast away on.

To a lesser degree, this kind of overcontrol is not all that unusual today; many children fit into a highly organized lifestyle that is dictated by their parents and their parents' needs, rather than by the child's needs, style, or wishes.

It happened that the father in the above case was a successful pediatrician. When asked if there was any correlation between sugar-coated cereal at age eight and health problems such as diabetes later in life, he said no. Yet when it came to outlawing sugar-coated cereal in his house, he could offer no valid explanation.

Several recommendations were made to this family. First was that they be more relaxed about food. Calcium is important for all children, but it can be obtained from other dairy products besides milk as well as from other foods, including vegetables and fish. Next, they were advised to allow for some spontaneity and "down time" in their lives—every week or so to go out together for pizza or ice cream, just for the fun of it. In addition, it was recommended that the eight-year-old should have an allowance of her own to do with as she pleased, and be given options for enjoying her free time, including watching television.

By the time this girl is fifteen, we'd like to see her enjoy a candy bar not as an expression of rebellious anger toward her mother or father, but because it is something she likes and deserves as a treat to herself.

As this case illustrates, many well-meaning parents take food and rules far too seriously for a child's own good. There is nothing wrong with parents' wanting more for a child than they had as children, if that is the goal, but such a goal can only be invested in a very few areas without a child's experiencing it as control, and not affection. Rules for children should be thought through carefully and logically, in each case asking, What *really* is the purpose? How serious are the consequences if the rule is not followed?

Fortunately, food is a very safe and easy area in which to relax the rules and, eventually, it is an area in which rules don't matter anyway. As children get older, issues such as white bread versus whole wheat bread, or soda versus fruit juice, become obsolete in the face of far more critical areas in which parental attention and guidance are essential, such as drinking and driving, sex and AIDS, and perhaps achieving reasonable expectations at school.

In addition to setting rules and standards, there is another, quite common way that we see the overcontrol of food backfire, involving parents who feel they have somehow "slipped up" if they give their child certain foods, or have failed if the family does not always have meals together or "on time." Perhaps this way of thinking is tied to guilt over not being a "good" parent—for example, feeling as if one is not as available to children as one would like to be due to economic pressures, career goals, or some other factor. Whatever the reason, when parents equate the feeding of a child with their own success as caregivers, children who do not fulfill these expectations pay a price. Teased, bribed, cajoled, or criticized, many of them learn as early as toddler age that their actions at mealtime can attract parental attention and elicit reactions; they begin to see food and feeding as opportunities to exercise control over the family, a state that can only increase tension and erupt into fights.

In the long run, these issues involving control are of far more concern than any health considerations here and now, or foods in this meal or the next. Schedules, food preferences, and eating patterns inevitably change. Parents should not feel bad if they cannot get their child to eat a good breakfast; if they give out snacks on demand or allow candy bars; serve macaroni and cheese every night for dinner because that's all their child wants to eat. When seen over the course of childhood and within the context of a varied diet, there is nothing intrinsically wrong with any of these foods, anyway.

What Should I Feed My Kids? is not a call to arms against nutritious food. It is a call to parents to put the issue of food in its proper perspective in relation to what is in the long-term best interests of the child. With this goal in mind, we hope our book will clarify food issues and misconceptions that cause tension in families—and help reverse the trend, however well intentioned, toward overcontrolling food. Beyond the time it takes to read this book, we believe matters concerning food should occupy no more that 5 percent of the time you and your child spend together.

Yes, there is room for parental guidance in encouraging children to make healthy food choices and to establish better eating patterns, but unless a child is on a medically regimented diet or substantially off his or her normal growth curve (see page 271), we see no reason to label foods as "safe" or "harmful" or to earmark specific foods for children to avoid completely in their diet. Despite what you read, none of the evidence, good or bad, linking food to health during adult years has been proven conclusively.

In his book, *The Hurried Child*, David Elkind argues that children are overstressed when treated like adults, that our adult model should not be their model. He urges parents not to rush children into assuming stressful adult situations, or to make demands on them that relate to an adult sense of achievement. In this book we want to urge parents not to hurry their children into taking on the adult view of food, either. Parents who can differentiate between their perceptions and needs regarding food and their child's can go far in avoiding unnecessary stress and conflict. We hope our book will help parents confidently recognize, accept, and embrace those differences.

Warning Signs of Overcontrol

Preoccupation with your child's diet—arguing with family members about meals and snacks; constantly discussing children's food; choosing what to do and where to go based on the quality of food that will be served.

Preoccupation with your own diet—becoming overly attentive to food and diet, which can set the stage for becoming overly attentive to a child's food and diet.

Food games, food bribes—trying to manipulate people at the dinner table to eat certain foods; playing one food against the other, such as withholding dessert until other foods are eaten.

Rigid rule making—basing rules on personal bias for or against certain foods rather than providing a fair, neutral ground for a child's choice making; enforcing rules by saying, "Because I said so," a sign that food is not the only issue involved.

Fifteen Good Reasons
Why You Can Let Them Eat Cake

Our basic philosophy is represented by these key points, expanded on in the chapters that follow.

1. *Growth proves that a child is getting the food he or she needs, not what's served in this meal or the next.* Measuring a child's growth involves more than just inches in length or quality of food. It includes the ability to make friends and master skills, to feel competent and proud of accomplishments. In other words, healthy growth includes well-rounded development.

2. *Food is not a life-or-death issue for children.* Normal adult concerns such as weight maintenance, low cholesterol, or fiber intake are not significant issues for children.

One of the reasons adults are so interested in food is that

they think it influences their life span or mortality in some way. What they think is harmful for them to eat they also think is harmful for their children, and yet there is no clear proof that what a person eats in childhood will help prevent disease and death later on. What we eat as adults can clearly affect our long-term health. A lower-fat diet appears to reduce the risk of heart disease or, in some cases, reverse established heart disease. It is also recognized that people who eat less food when they are older—and particularly in the latter third of their life—increase their chance of living longer, although no one knows why.

Unless there are true health problems as determined by a pediatrician, there is no reason why any child needs to overly restrict fat, cholesterol, salt, sugar, or anything else in his or her diet.

3. *Children's nutritional requirements are different from adults'.* They are not trying to control or maintain an optimum weight; they are increasing it. When an adult reaches midlife, body metabolism begins to slow down. To stay in shape, adults must lower the quantities of food they eat and increase physical activity. In contrast, a child's metabolism is geared to growth and, in comparison with most adults, a very active life-style. Growth and activity require lots of energy. To deprive children of certain foods—any one particular food or many foods—is not only unnecessary but, in terms of good growth and health, may even deprive them of the energy and vitamin stores they need, especially during infancy and adolescence, when growth is accelerated.

4. *There are only two phases of childhood in which growth is intense and the need for energy-rich or high-calorie food is great—infancy and puberty.* In the middle-childhood years (ages two to ten, approximately) growth slows down and nutrition requirements can be eased. In other words, for the majority of childhood, parents need not pressure children or worry about every meal they eat or its effect on growth.

5. *"Good eating habits" are not fixed for life in childhood.* The

idea that, "It's up to me to teach good eating habits early on or she'll never learn to eat well," is detrimental in that it unnecessarily puts pressure on parent and child. There is no evidence that forcing children to eat certain foods or forbidding others will result in "better" or "worse" eating habits later on. As it does with children who are pressured to attain a high level of achievement in school, insisting on "good eating habits" may also backfire. If food becomes too major a part of the parent-child relationship—for example, overly controlled or seen as a life-or-death issue—it may contribute to long-term emotional problems that can include symptoms such as eating disorders.

6. *Food is not the only determinant of a child's growth and appearance.* Heredity may factor as much as 60 to 80 percent into how much body fat a person carries, and in whether a youngster is tall, short, thin, or big boned. Environment also makes a contribution, particularly the influence of parental life-style, exercise, and family dietary habits. Patterns of poor eating or constant dieting by parents may determine much of children's food intake during the time they are living at home, while their preference for a sensible diet will emerge when they are on their own.

7. *Exercise and fitness are pursued differently by children than they are by adults.* Adults equate exercise and fitness with sports, gym equipment, or working out in front of an exercise video. Children, largely through daily activity, pursue them simply for fun. Despite statistics that show children becoming increasingly unfit and their life-styles more sedentary than in the past, most children run around during much of their day, often when their parents do not see them. So unless there is real evidence on the growth chart that an individual child is off his or her curve, there is no need to treat the child as a population statistic and worry that the child is too sedentary, or try to push him or her into an exercise program.

8. *Erratic eating is normal in children, reflecting behaviors that typify a child's stage of development.* Appetite levels and food

preferences are changing all the time in children, as are the quantity and kind of food they will eat. All of this is acceptable. Bizarre as they may seem to you, monotonous or unappealing food preferences are perfectly normal, and in time (perhaps as early as the next meal), will change.

9. *A child's natural appetite cues him or her on when to eat. The child knows best whether he or she is hungry or full.* Prodded, coerced, or held back from eating, children soon lose touch with their natural appetite cues. That can lead to overeating. Children at an early age benefit from feeding themselves and choosing what they want from the food their parents make available. Making a variety of nutritious foods available and outlawing nothing is also one of the best and safest ways for parents who tend to be too controlling to practice letting go.

10. *"Picky eating" at one meal can be made up for with a healthy snack later or good food at the next meal.* Given a wide choice of foods for snacks and meals over the course of a day or a few days, the vast majority of children more than meet their nutritional requirements and stay right along their growth curve. They get just as much nutrition out of snacks as they do out of meals.

11. *Vitamin deficiencies affecting growth are very rare in children.* As it can create stress among parents, the concept of the "required daily allowance" (RDA) is important to understand. These recommended amounts for daily consumption are deliberately set at a high level, taking into account that different people on different diets will absorb only a percentage of the vitamins and minerals in their food. The RDA is set to overcompensate for these differences without putting anyone in danger of having too much of the nutrient—a kind of "maximum safe allowance." However, it is very unlikely that anyone consuming even 50 percent of the RDA of a certain nutrient will become deficient in that nutrient.

12. *There is no food that can be specified as "bad."* Good nutrition for children results from easy access to all kinds of foods within the framework of a balanced diet. Despite all the

theories on how to ensure good health and nutrition—and some people say "enforcement" or restriction is the only way—we concur with the opinion of the American Academy of Pediatrics and the American Dietetic Association that no food is "bad," and that no food should be on the forbidden list.

13. *Sugar does not cause hyperactivity or inattention in children; chocolate does not create insomnia.* These are two common misconceptions that have grown out of the need that some adults have to outlaw good-tasting food. Other controversies that cause confusion about food choices include the use of additives and artificial ingredients, the place of "junk food" in a child's diet, and the influence of television on their preferences. These are important issues for parents to resolve, and are covered in the first part of this book.

14. *Deprivation heightens desire.* Children who have been restricted in what they eat eventually find ways to get forbidden foods—at birthday parties, through trading lunches, with allowance—and they go after those foods with special intensity.

15. *Food is a very safe area for children to learn to exercise choice.* Sharing meals and snacks is a great way to enjoy "down time" together—to enjoy, rather than judge, food choices.

Everyday Applications: The First Steps to Eliminating Food Stress

- *Show some flexibility in your view of what your child chooses to eat.* Do not get hung up on the quality of this meal or that, or equate your child's eating style or choices of food with his or her health. Review food intake over the course of several days or a week—not on the basis of one meal or one day's worth of foods. Take the long-term view. The pattern of growth is the key, not one day's or even one month's food or eating patterns.
- *When you find yourself in a fight over food, stop.* What

should you realistically expect of your child? If you feel tension over food—for example, you begin to think your child will die unless he or she follows your rules—or if food choices take on a life-or-death quality, there may be issues from your own life involving the need for control that have nothing to do with nutrition.

- *Allocate to food and food issues no more than 5 percent of time with your child.*
- *Offer a wide variety of nutritious foods and make them part of a varied, well-balanced diet.* As for quantities of food eaten, let children make that determination.
- *Outlaw nothing.* Unless you or your child is on a medically restricted diet, do not treat any one food as "good" or "bad," "healthy" or "junk."
- *Show tolerance.* When you read terms like *carageenan* or *guar gum* on a label, don't jump to the conclusion that these ingredients are bad just because you don't know what they are. A better approach to take is exemplified by the story that appeared in the news about how tolerance of ethnic groups had increased. Pollsters asked participants to rank various ethnic groups for their acceptability (Norwegians, Anglo-Saxons, Germans, Koreans, etc.), among whom they included a fictitious group, the Wisians. Sixty-one percent of those who participated in the poll showed tolerance of the Wisians by withholding their ranking until they had more information. They gave Wisians the benefit of the doubt.

In similar fashion, don't rule out a specific food until you know more about it, or restrict or increase certain foods in the family diet because of what you hear in the news. Get more information first.

- *Don't give up when foods are rejected.* Keep offering them. Children's eating patterns change.
- *Do not expect more "healthy eating" from your child than you do from yourself.* In other words, check your own eating patterns and don't be hypocritical. Do you snack

on ice cream at midnight and expect your child not to have a dessert? Do you have a big lunch, and then expect your child, who may not have had a big lunch, to have a simple supper with you?

- *Don't let your own commitment to nutrition get in the way of your child's friendships or fun.* Is he or she invited out after school for pizza? Great! There's nothing bad about pizza nutritionally; being part of a group of friends having fun is more important. Was there a birthday party at school with candy bars or cupcakes? Again, your child was sharing good times with friends. Don't add an overlay of guilt to the child's fun by giving condescending looks if he or she had soda or treats you never have at home. If a party invitation arrives in your house and you hear, "Oh boy, chocolate cake!" rather than, "Oh boy, so-and-so's birthday party!" take it as your cue that food is too important in your house and it's time to let up.

- *Don't forget you were once a child, enjoying foods you probably don't eat now.* French fries and a Coke; hot fudge sundaes after school; bubble gum and cotton candy— these foods trigger enjoyable memories for many adults today. Let your child discover his or her own childish food preferences, building memories he or she, too, will remember fondly as an adult.

◆　　◆　　◆

The
Controversies

1

❖ ❖ ❖ ❖

Is It Safe?
Pesticides, Additives,
and Food Risks

The question of whether pesticide residues or additives are harmful to children is a valid one, but these risks are often exaggerated while the dangers of food-borne illnesses, such as salmonella, are underplayed or ignored.

Clearly, the issue of food safety needs to be placed in a balanced perspective. As this chapter will show, there are many ways to do that—from becoming an educated consumer who understands the role of pesticides and additives in foods, to practicing safe handling, cooking, and storage at home.

Pesticide Risks and Benefits

Pesticides were developed to control plant and pest diseases that threaten crops, food supplies, and ultimately human health. As with many other solutions to human health problems, such as X rays and medications, there is some risk involved in pesticide use but that does not cancel out their benefits. Even essential nutrients like vitamins and minerals can be toxic in high doses.

One approach to pesticides is to avoid them completely. Before going to this extreme, however, consider the following:

- Health authorities such as the U.S. Centers for Disease Control, the Food and Drug Administration (FDA), and the American Cancer Society confirm that the health benefits of eating fruits and vegetables far outweigh any potential risks associated with dietary exposure to pesticides. For adults, fruits and vegetables reduce the risk of cancer and other chronic diseases, and they contribute to better health. The vitamins and minerals in fruits and vegetables contribute to the child's daily needs for good growth and development.

- Foods in the "all-natural" category may contain harmful molds or bacteria that, without the use of pesticides or preservatives, are difficult to control or eradicate, or may lead to the early spoilage of food. As an example, raw "natural honey" may contain botulinum spores that could cause a fatal infection in young infants.

In 1990, under the auspices of the Institute of Food Technologists, a group of food experts from fourteen professional societies representing more than 100,000 scientists convened to evaluate the overall safety of the food supply and to rank their major areas of concern. In marked contrast to current consumer perceptions, these scientists overwhelmingly ranked contamination from microbes and naturally occurring toxins in foods as their major areas of concern. In serving the population at large, it appears that one of the most effective ways to reduce the risk of contamination is through the carefully regulated mass production of foods—as witnessed by the American Dietetic Association's report that over 70 percent of botulism outbreaks have been traced to home-canned or home-processed foods, and only 9 percent to commercial food sources.

• Rigid testing standards are geared to establish safe exposures to additives and pesticides, taking into account the special needs and dietary patterns of children who tend to eat more fruits and vegetables than adults.

• Most scientists agree that children are not necessarily at increased risk with pesticides, and in some cases they may be at less risk than adults.

In assessing both short- and long-term risks of pesticide use, each substance is evaluated by the FDA and other food-regulating agencies to judge toxicity and safety.

Pesticides are subjected to more than 120 separate tests involving how they work and how they affect humans, fish, wildlife, and the environment. After an approval process that takes up to ten years to complete, only about one in twenty thousand new pesticide products makes it from the lab to the farmer's field.

• The "maximum tolerance dose" (MTD) of pesticides used on foods is normally thousands of times more than what could typically be present in our diet, while the residual pesticides amount allowed in the human diet is also one hundred to a thousand times lower than the levels established in safety tests involving laboratory animals. Recent recommendations from the National Academy of Sciences should help the FDA to become even better at assessing any risk that might be unique to infants or children from pesticides.

• The FDA is continually measuring detectable residues in common grocery-shelf foods. Residues detected are usually far below established standards.

• For personal reassurance, routinely washing fruits and vegetables with plain water will remove any residues that may exist.

Food Additives

A food additive is broadly defined as any substance added to food—the most common being sugar, salt, and corn syrup. Without additives, ice cream would form icy crystals, peanut butter would separate, and marshmallows would be hard.

As with pesticides, the use of food additives is also highly regulated. In 1959, the FDA established the GRAS list (Generally Recognized As Safe). This followed the 1958 passage of the Delaney Clause, an amendment to the Food, Drug and Cosmetic Act stating that *no additive known to cause cancer in animals or humans may be put into food in any amount.* Any new additive has to be approved before it can be marketed. The manufacturer must convince the FDA through rigorous testing that the additive is effective and does not cause cancer or birth defects.

When the testing is completed, the FDA reviews the results and invites public response to the manufacturer's petition for acceptance of the new additive. If approval is given, the FDA establishes regulations for the types of foods in which the additive can be used, the maximum quantities that can be used, and how the substance must be described on the label. Additives in foods are limited to no more than 1/100th of the amount that was found safe for test animals.

When an additive is proposed for use in meat or poultry products, it must also be approved by the U.S. Department of Agriculture's Food Safety Inspection Service (FSIS), which applies different standards that take into account the unique characteristics of meat and poultry products. For example, FSIS would not allow the use of sorbic acid, an approved additive, in meat salads because it could mask spoilage.

- Except for a small number of reactions that occur in people with specific allergies, there are very few documented cases of harm from additives. Additives play a minor role, if any, in hyperactivity. A study by the National

Institutes of Health showed that very few hyperactive children benefit from an additive-free diet. In fact, one of the primary uses of additives is to protect food quality and safety—for example, to maintain and improve nutritional value; keep foods fresh; slow microbial growth and prevent spoilage; give desired texture, flavor, and appearance; and aid in processing and preparation.

- Regulation has greatly reduced the use of color additives in food. In 1960, there were nearly two hundred colors used in foods; in 1989, only thirty-three were approved for use by the FDA. Their use includes ensuring uniformity of color; giving an attractive appearance to foods that would otherwise be unappetizing; and helping protect flavor and light-sensitive vitamins in foods during storage.

Consumers can choose foods with or without additives. If food-related allergies are present, a careful reading of labels will determine whether foods contain ingredients that cause sensitivity in some individuals. These foods can be limited or avoided.

IF YOU WISH TO LIMIT FOOD ADDITIVES:

- Plan meals around fresh fruits and vegetables.
- Limit intake of packaged and highly processed convenience foods.
- Use fresh meat or poultry products instead of processed meats such as cold cuts.
- Read ingredient lists on food labels.

SPECIAL CONCERNS

BST and IGF-1 A furor has arisen over a genetically engineered hormone that is identical to a natural, milk-producing hormone in cows—BST (bovine somatotropin). Synthetic BST boosts milk production in low-producing cows by 10 to 15 percent.

Certain advocacy groups have warned that synthetic BST in milk will bring it to dangerous levels in humans, wreck havoc with human hormones, or cause health problems in cows. None of these effects has been proven. Samples of milk from cows treated with synthetic BST reveal the same amount of the hormone as is found in milk from untreated cows. Nutrients are found in equal amounts in both. BST—whether synthetic or natural—is inactive in humans; it cannot stimulate milk production or anything else because the human body does not recognize it as a hormone.

Problems with cows treated with BST have also been exaggerated. Increased milk production was feared to lead to more cases of mastitis in cows and thus to an increase of antibiotics in the milk supply. But milk is constantly tested for antibiotics and, if so much as a trace is found, the milk is discarded and farmers lose money.

Another BST-related concern involves IGF-1 (insulin-like growth factor 1), a natural hormone stimulated by BST and used by cows and humans for healthy cell growth, for example, in the formation of the liver. Advertisements have stated that IGF-1 causes cells to divide and therefore may be responsible for causing tumors. This is a scare tactic. IGF-1 is found in human milk and saliva; the growth it induces is normal organ growth, and there is no evidence it is responsible for tumors.

The efforts by some consumer advocacy groups to protect the public against these genetically engineered products seem to us and many others to be misguided. Whether the United States needs more milk or not is irrelevant. BST is one of the first of the applications of genetic engineering to improve the nutritional quality or quantity of our food supply, and it has the potential to be of great value where milk and dairy products are in short supply.

Nitrates and Nitrites Through a lack of information or a tendency to interpret the worst, consumers frequently overemphasize the harmful effects of these naturally occurring chemicals.

Nitrate and nitrite are similar compounds consisting of nitrogen with three oxygen molecules (nitrate), or nitrogen with two oxygen molecules (nitrite). These chemicals are a natural component of some of the foods we eat, and also became part of our diet through the use of fertilizers and preservatives. They occur in nature through the action of bacteria on organic matter in the soil, and are found in ground water as well as in plants and living matter that grow in the soil. They are also found in fertilizers that contain nitrogen, an essential chemical found in all proteins. When those fertilizers enter ground water or well water, they can increase the concentration of nitrates or nitrites in the human diet.

The largest percentage of nitrates and nitrites in the typical human diet—about 70 percent—comes from vegetables, in particular cauliflower, spinach, broccoli, and root vegetables such as potatoes and carrots. Another 20 percent comes from drinking water, and the remaining 5 to 10 percent comes from meat and meat products in which sodium nitrate is used as a preservative and color-enhancing agent.

Risks and Benefits. Because they are ubiquitous, the presence of nitrates in the diet is unavoidable, yet the amount found in most commercially prepared foods is not something parents need to be concerned about. The risk of cancer from these compounds is nil, and the risk of poisoning leading to insufficient oxygen (cyanosis) or respiratory distress is very rare. In the world's literature, there have been about two thousand cases reported over the past fifty years, often from rural areas.

Both human and experimental animal studies have failed to provide conclusive evidence that nitrate or nitrite ingestion causes either carcinogenic effects or serious malformations. While some of the nitrates in the diet can go on to form nitrosamines, compounds some of which are carcinogens, most of them are absorbed and metabolized into harmless compounds or just excreted in the stool. Cancer-causing nitrosamines can be avoided in the diet by lowered cooking temperatures of processed foods, particularly bacon, and by avoiding the use of rendered bacon fat in cooking. Eating bacon will *not* cause cancer.

As for benefits, used as a preservative in processed foods nitrates preserve color, prevent spoilage, and inhibit the growth of the bacteria that produce botulinum toxin, a potentially deadly poison.

Sulfites Five to 10 percent of persons with asthma may be sensitive to sulfites and their reactions can be severe. Sulfites are used to maintain a fresh appearance in produce and to stop light-colored fruits and vegetables from darkening. The FDA requires labels on foods that contain sulfites; the use of sulfites on salad bar ingredients was banned in 1986. Processed potatoes, many dried fruits, and some beer and wine contain sulfites.

MSG Monosodium glutamate is a common flavor enhancer. Although it has been judged safe for use by adults, it should be avoided by infants, pregnant women, and persons who are sensitive to it. Symptoms of intolerance include a flushed face, chest pain, and a throbbing headache that occur about twenty minutes after eating MSG.

FD&C Yellow #5, or Tartrazine This food color causes an allergic reaction in one or two out of every ten thousand people. Symptoms include hives, itching, and nasal congestion. People allergic to aspirin are most likely to be affected. FD&C Yellow #5 is often in orange drinks, gelatin, cake mixes, processed cheese dinners, and snacks. When tartrazine is used in a food product, the label must state its presence.

Food Safety at Home

Learning how to handle food at home is one of the easiest ways to eliminate preventable illnesses, such as salmonella poisoning and other bacterial risks, that result from contamination of food. The major cause of food contamination is improper preparation, cooking, and storage of food, which allow germs to grow and multiply. Given sufficient time and the right conditions, harmful bacteria can spread:

- in cooked food left to cool on the counter;
- in frozen food left to thaw outside the refrigerator;
- at buffet tables where food is kept at unsafe temperatures;
- in undercooked meats and poultry;
- on soiled cutting boards;
- on utensils that go from job to job without being washed.

To avoid problems, practice these three rules in the kitchen:

1. *Keep food clean.* Among other sanitation measures, wash your hands frequently while preparing food; use clean towels, sponges, cooking dishes, and utensils; scrub counters and sanitize cutting boards between food preparation steps; let cleaned utensils and cutting boards air dry.

2. *Keep hot food hot.* All cooked foods should be cooked and held at temperatures higher than 140 degrees F. High temperatures (165 to 212 degrees F.) kill most bacteria. Lower cooking and holding temperatures prevent growth but may let bacteria survive.

3. *Keep cold food cold.* All cooked foods that are to be served cold and stored should be rapidly cooled to 40 degrees F. or below. At this temperature, only slow growth of certain spoilage bacteria can occur. Below 32 degrees (freezing) some bacteria may survive but won't grow.

REFRIGERATING TIPS

- Leave food in store wrapping unless the wrapping is torn. The less you handle food, the better.
- Keep all foods wrapped or in covered containers.
- Store food in small portions in shallow dishes for faster cooling.

- Make sure storage containers seal tightly, to prevent moisture loss.

FREEZING TIPS

- Keep foods purchased frozen in their original packaging.
- Rewrap other food carefully, using freezer containers, foils, and moisture-proof paper or other wraps. Freezer tape helps ensure airtightness and eliminate freezer burn. (While not harmful, freezer burn will make food tough and tasteless.)
- Organize your freezer with oldest foods to the front so they will be used first. Label each package with item, date, and number of servings.
- Be cautious about refreezing partially thawed food. Food to be refrozen must still have ice crystals on it, and have only been in the refrigerator for one day or less. As quality may be lost with refreezing, consider cooking the food well before refreezing it.

COLD STORAGE GUIDELINES

Install a thermometer inside both the refrigerator and freezer. Periodically check the temperatures. Set refrigerator between 34 and 40 degrees F. Set freezer at 0 degrees or lower, never above 5 degrees F.

SAFETY TIPS FOR CANNED FOODS

- Keep the cupboard or pantry clean, dry, dark, and cool. Ideal storage temperatures are between 40 and 70 degrees F. High temperatures (over 100) are harmful to canned goods.
- Organize the cupboard with older cans up front for earlier use (canned goods generally keep for at least one year).
- Be alert for signs of spoilage. Never use food from cans that are cracked, bulging, or leaking, or that spurt liquid

Food	Refrigerator	Freezer
Bacon	7 days	1 month
Beef roast	3 to 4 weeks	6 to 12 months
Butter	1 to 2 weeks	6 to 9 months
Chicken, raw	1 to 2 days	9 to 12 months
Chicken, cooked	1 to 4 days	4 to 6 months
Eggs, fresh	4 to 5 weeks	——
Eggs, hard cooked	1 week	——
Ham	3 to 7 days	1 to 2 months
Hamburger	1 to 2 days	2 to 3 months
Hot dogs, unopened	check package date or 14 days	1 to 2 months
Hot dogs, opened	7 days	1 to 2 months
Lean fish	1 to 2 days (iced); 1 day (uniced)	6 months
Lunch meats (cold cuts)	3 to 5 days after vacuum seal is broken; 2 weeks if sealed in original packaging	1 to 2 months
Margarine	1 to 2 weeks	4 to 6 months
Meats, cooked	3 to 4 days	2 to 3 months
Pork chops	2 to 3 days	3 to 4 months
Pork or veal roast	2 to 3 days	4 to 8 months

when opened. Don't taste! These spoilage signs may indicate the presence of the deadly bacteria that cause botulism. Discard these cans immediately.

SAFE FOOD-HANDLING TIPS
FOR PARENTS AND CHILDREN

• Wash hands thoroughly with soap and water before and after handling food (especially after diapering, playing, or working with young children).
• Wash all work surfaces, utensils, and your hands immediately after they have come in contact with raw meat, raw fish, raw poultry, or raw eggs. Never let any raw juices from these foods touch any other food, or remain on kitchen utensils.
• Thoroughly scrub cutting boards immediately after use with hot soapy water, or clean them in the dishwasher.

- Avoid serving raw fish (i.e., sushi, oysters, clams) or dishes made with raw eggs that could contain harmful bacteria, viruses, or parasites.
- Avoid using cracked eggs or serving foods that contain raw eggs. If cookie, bread, or cake dough contains raw eggs, don't lick the bowl or spoon. In homemade ice cream recipes that call for raw egg yolks, use an egg substitute that has been pasteurized or follow a recipe that calls for cooking the ice cream mixture before freezing. (Use egg substitutes whenever uncooked eggs are part of a recipe—for example, in homemade mayonnaise, chocolate mousse, etc.)
- Thaw meats and poultry in your refrigerator overnight or in a microwave oven. If thawed in a microwave, cook immediately. Never thaw meats on the counter at room temperature.
- Use a meat thermometer to check internal temperature of oven-cooked foods. Be sure to follow microwave directions, rotating dishes and allowing standing time if required. Check internal food temperature in a variety of areas. Cook poultry and pork until well done.
- Keep hot foods above 140 degrees F. and cold foods below 40 degrees F. Do not allow foods to sit at room temperature for more than two hours. Bacteria multiply fastest between 40 and 140 degrees F.
- Store leftover canned food in an airtight container in the refrigerator. Remove leftover stuffing from poultry and store separately.
- Cool leftovers quickly in the refrigerator or freezer. Large batches should be divided into small portions in shallow containers so food can cool more quickly. To allow air to circulate, do not stack items during cooling or freezing. Reheat leftovers to at least 165 degrees F.
- Do not save raw or cooked food too long (see table, page 27). Food permeated with harmful bacteria does not necessarily have a foul odor or spoiled appearance.

2

◆ ◆ ◆ ◆

Cholesterol, Fat, and Children

For children especially, cholesterol and fat must be seen first and foremost for their contribution to good health. Both are essential for healthy body metabolism, particularly during periods of active growth and development, when energy (calorie) needs are high.

Cholesterol, a waxy chemical that is manufactured in the liver, is essential for the body's proper functioning. It helps build new cells and repair old ones. It acts as a building block for the brain, nerves, internal organs, and several hormones found naturally in the human body. It is utilized by the body to produce many essential substances—for example, bile, which aids in digestion.

Fat, which is found in both plants and animals, is used by the body as a concentrated source of energy, permitting relatively small, infrequent amounts of food to be eaten while obtaining the calories necessary to maintain daily activities. It is also utilized by the body in other ways—for example, in the normal functioning of the immune system, and in growth.

It is important to emphasize that *in reasonable amounts (see below), fat helps a child grow to his or her full potential.* Moreover, excessive restriction of dietary fat in the early childhood years has been shown to cause growth failure among children and adolescents.

The three main fats included in the human diet are referred to as saturated, polyunsaturated, and monounsaturated. Saturated fats, which tend to raise the blood's cholesterol level, come from animals and some plants and are solid at room temperature. Examples include beef fat and coconuts.

Polyunsaturated fats, for example, corn oil and safflower oil, are usually liquid at room temperature and help lower the blood's cholesterol level.

Monounsaturated fats, such as canola and olive oil, are also liquid and are usually obtained from vegetables. Research suggests that monounsaturated fats are as effective as polyunsaturated oils in decreasing blood cholesterol levels.

Why All the Fuss about Cholesterol and Fat?

Only a small percentage of cholesterol in the body comes from food—about 20 percent in comparison with about 80 percent produced by the body. However, certain foods, specifically those containing large amounts of saturated fat, discourage the body from clearing away excess cholesterol, the buildup of which accounts for the cautionary approach to fat in the diet. When cholesterol does build up in the arteries, it can block the supply of blood to the heart, making it more difficult for the heart to nourish itself. This can result in a heart attack.

Although no one knows exactly why certain people have heart attacks, there is a correlation between the *risk* of having a heart attack and the amount of cholesterol in one's bloodstream, which varies from individual to individual, depending on genetic makeup and the ability to utilize or remove unneeded cholesterol efficiently (this ability also varies among individuals). In the presence of certain other factors—for example, obesity, heavy smoking, heavy drinking, a sedentary life-style, a genetic pattern of heart attacks in the family—a continuously high blood cholesterol level has been shown to increase the risk of heart attacks in adults. For this reason, doctors watch cholesterol levels more closely in susceptible adults. If their cholesterol is high, it suggests that excess amounts *may* be accumulating in the arteries, rather than being transported out of the body. (However, it is important to note that a high cholesterol reading does not indicate *definite* accumulations.)

THE LDL FACTOR

Cholesterol takes a long time to accumulate and cause problems, and as recent information has shown, much of the risk has to do with the efficiency of the cholesterol transport system in an individual. Cholesterol is transported in the blood by two kinds of protein molecules—low-density lipoproteins (LDL) and high-density lipoproteins (HDL). The LDL molecules deposit cholesterol into the body through the bloodstream; the HDL molecules carry it out. These two components make up one's "total cholesterol," which, to be considered safe, should register at or below 200 mg/dl for an adult. The ratio of LDL to HDL cholesterol is a better indicator of possible risk of heart or circulatory problems than one's total cholesterol. Too much LDL cholesterol and/or too little HDL cholesterol may be associated with an overload of cholesterol being deposited and remaining in the arteries, including the coronary arteries (blood vessels that supply the heart muscle). In other words, for adults the higher the LDL number, the higher the cardiac risk.*

The blood-testing procedures upon which current knowl-

---

*An LDL cholesterol above 110 mg/dl and/or an HDL cholesterol below 50 put one at increased risk for heart disease.

edge of cholesterol metabolism is based are a boon to adults who may be susceptible to heart disease. By lowering total cholesterol—both by reducing the intake of foods that contain cholesterol and saturated fat and by regular exercise—these individuals may reduce the risk of accumulating cholesterol in their circulatory system.

At the same time, these indicators and sophisticated testing methods have fueled controversy and confusion over whether to measure cholesterol levels in children.

All Children Do Not Need Testing

The prevailing view of cholesterol in children is that (1) you've got to measure it, (2) if it's high you've got to do something about it, and (3) if you don't do something about it, the child is certain to have a heart attack when he or she becomes an adult. In our opinion, and that of many others, this view is oversimplified. The accumulation of cholesterol in the arteries occurs over a lifetime. The ability to tell someone, especially a child, that he or she is definitely going to suffer some consequences is scientifically without basis at this time. Not all those with "high cholesterols" are going to end up with clogged arteries. In spite of all the concern about heart attacks, they are extremely rare before the age of forty, even in those with blood cholesterols of 200 to 240 mg/dl. What is quite certain is that there are harmful effects of overemphasizing cholesterol-lowering nutrition—that is, making cholesterol a bigger issue for a child than it should be, which can cause unnecessary stress for him or her.

Therefore, in concurrence with the views held by the American Academy of Pediatrics and the National Cholesterol Education Program, it is our opinion that all children should not be routinely tested for cholesterol. Although some experts do maintain that all children should have their blood cholesterol tested regularly, the arguments against this approach are compelling:

- Fifty percent of children with high cholesterol levels do not end up in the high-risk (aggressive treatment) category as young adults.
- Blood cholesterol tests do not identify with certainty which children are going to grow up to develop heart disease. The link between the risk of heart disease and an elevated blood cholesterol is well established in adults but this risk has not been well established for children.
- Labeling children as being at risk for heart disease may be harmful, particularly if it leads to unnecessary diet restrictions or to the use of cholesterol-lowering medications.
- Lipid-lowering drugs have the potential for interfering with growth as well as producing other significant side effects.
- The process of atherosclerosis (hardening of the arteries) occurs slowly, even if it does begin in childhood and adolescence. Blockage of the blood vessels to the heart usually takes fifty to sixty years to develop. The optimal time for aggressive intervention is not yet certain, but it clearly depends on identifying accurately those who are truly going to develop coronary artery disease, particularly at an early age. We know that it is possible to significantly reverse coronary artery disease even at age forty or fifty. Perhaps, then, treatment efforts should begin after age twenty, when growth and development are completed and the risks of intervention can be minimized.
- Recommended dietary guidelines serve everyone, tested or untested and including those children considered high risk, for whom they serve as safe initial intervention.

Whom to Test? Determining Who Is at Risk

The National Cholesterol Education Program (NCEP), an expert panel of physicians, nutritionists, and heart specialists, has issued their guidelines for identifying children in this country at risk for heart disease and what should be done to minimize the risk. In their estimate, children and adolescents at risk include those who:

- have a family history (parents or grandparents) of cardio-vascular disease or heart attack, stroke, or peripheral vascular disease occurring before age fifty-five;
- have at least one parent who has a high blood cholesterol reading (over 240 mg/dl);
- have a normal family history or family history on record but who are obese, have high blood pressure, and/or smoke cigarettes.

If these risk factors for elevated cholesterol have been identified, then cholesterol screening may be warranted, as advised by the family doctor. However, children should not be tested for cholesterol earlier than age two, except in rare circumstances.

Evaluating Test Results

The National Cholesterol Education Program's recommendations for cholesterol levels in children are as follows:

Category	Total Cholesterol	LDL Cholesterol
Acceptable	less than 170 mg/dl	less than 110 mg/dl
Borderline	170 to 199 mg/dl	110 to 129 mg/dl
High	200 mg/dl or more	130 mg/dl or more

If a child's cholesterol is tested and the total is found to be over 170 mg/dl, then the test should be repeated within one month. If the total cholesterol remains beyond 170 mg/dl, then the child's LDL cholesterol level should be tested. If the LDL cholesterol is greater than 110 mg/dl, the child and parents should be educated about a prudent diet.

Those children with a family history of early heart disease or strokes should have an LDL cholesterol level measured on the first screening.

For those children with over 130 mg/dl of LDL cholesterol, more intensive dietary counseling should be undertaken, and for children whose LDL cholesterol is 160 mg/dl or higher, more restrictive diets may be necessary.

Cholesterol-lowering medication is suggested only with children who in repeat tests and in the presence of risk factors indicated above are shown to have very elevated LDL cholesterol levels (over 190 mg/dl) and who are at least ten years of age. Some even recommend waiting until the child has stopped growing before starting drug treatment. (Drug therapy has been used with some younger children with exceptionally elevated LDL cholesterol levels, under very careful supervision by experts in blood lipid disorders.)

There are several points to keep in mind about cholesterol test results in children:

- The higher the reading, the more accurate the prediction that an individual is at risk. High readings in childhood, however, mainly serve to identify the individual who is at higher *risk* for heart disease as an adult; they do not predict who will actually develop it.
- Blood cholesterols in children tend to fluctuate, and they rise just before children go into puberty. This is normal, as hormones are changing and hormones affect blood cholesterol.
- Seventy-five percent of all children do not need their cholesterol levels tested and would come out with satisfactory levels (low to normal) if they did. However, satisfactory levels do not imply that diet should be ignored. Everyone should learn and follow the principles of good nutrition.

Dietary Guidelines and Applications

To help keep cholesterol and fat at healthy levels, the recommended guidelines as set forth by the American Academy of Pediatrics are:

1. Approximately 300 milligrams of cholesterol per day for children two years of age or older.

2. Total fat content approximately 30 percent of the diet— two thirds of which should be taken in as unsaturated fat, one third saturated. (See sample low-fat menus at the end of this chapter.)

Saturated Fats These are fats found in foods derived from plants and animals in varying degrees—highly marbleized meats such as bacon and "expensive" cuts of beef, butter, cream, whole milk, cheeses made from cream and whole milk, coconuts, and cashews, to name a few. High levels of saturated fat in the diet are what elevate blood cholesterol. One reason saturated fats may contribute to heart and vascular problems is that they interfere with the body's ability to scavenge excessive amounts of cholesterol from the blood.

Monounsaturated Fats These include vegetable oils such as canola oil and olive oil, and are part of a healthier diet.

Polyunsaturated Fats These include oils from vegetable products such as safflower and sunflower seeds, corn, soybeans, and cottonseeds. A balance of these fats, together with saturated and monounsaturated fats, are healthier for the body than a diet dominated by saturated or unsaturated fats. An excess amount of polyunsaturated fats in the diet has been linked to other health problems, such as the development of gallstones.

(Once again, none of these dietary recommendations should be applied to children from birth to two years of age, a period of rapid growth and development when restricting fat and cholesterol intake may have very serious consequences.)

APPLICATIONS

Early childhood can be seen as a transition period during which the fat and cholesterol content of the diet should gradually decrease to the recommended amounts. Actually, if you look at the normal weaning process, from the liquid diet to solid foods, you would see that this gradual process happens naturally. The infant diet of breast milk or infant formula contains approximately 50 percent of the calories from the milk fat content and, as solids are introduced during the first and second year of age, the percentage of fat calories decreases.

Sensible eating habits play the key role for everyone in how to approach dietary cholesterol.

All of us, including children over two years of age, should pay more attention to lowering the fat and cholesterol in our diets—for example, by using lower-fat cheese and low-fat milk instead of whole milk, and by eating lean meats.

However, while many of the adult dietary recommendations about a low-fat diet can be safely applied to children in preventing health problems, *it would be a mistake to overemphasize high cholesterol as a risk to most children as there is no way yet of precisely predicting who will have heart problems later in life.*

The primary goal of diet in childhood is to achieve normal growth and development; no child should be made to feel that he or she has a disease or that the child is at risk if he or she eats certain foods.

The best insurance against high cholesterol is a diet that offers a wide variety of foods that are low in saturated fats and cholesterol: lean meats and low-fat dairy products (critical sources of protein, iron, and calcium); vegetables, grains, and fruit—all included as part of a physically active, pleasurable life-style.

Familiarize yourself with the cholesterol and fat content of the foods your family eats, and use that information as *a general guideline* to be sure you are within recommended quotas over the course of a few days.

Can your child choose chocolate milk with lunch, if desired, or have an egg every other day? Of course. Chocolate milk is made with skim milk and chocolate flavoring; an egg has about 240 mg cholesterol, and is a good source of other nutrients. Both fit nicely into a varied meal plan for growing children.

No single food should be excluded from a child's diet for nutritional reasons. Even consumed several times a week, no single food will exceed recommended guidelines. In the total picture of a balanced diet, there is no good reason why ice cream should not be considered a good dessert!

Under 30 Percent of Calories from Fat— What a Day's Worth Looks Like

The following menus are not intended to recommend certain or specific foods but rather to illustrate "patterns" of food selection that over time lead to a nutritious, leaner diet.

Sample Low-Fat Menu for a Preschooler (Ages 2 to 5)
BREAKFAST:
- 4   ounces apple juice
- ¾   cup Cream of Wheat
- 4   ounces 1 percent milk (1 gram fat compared to 4 grams in whole milk)

SNACK:
- 2   squares graham crackers
- 4   ounces orange juice

LUNCH:
-    peanut butter and jelly sandwich
- 1 ½   tablespoons peanut butter

1   tablespoon jelly
     whole wheat bread
½   apple
4   ounces 1 percent milk
SNACK:
4   ounces low-fat yogurt (2 grams fat compared to almost 4
     grams in whole-milk yogurt)
DINNER:
2   ounces ham, lean
½   cup garden peas
½   cup mashed potatoes with 1 teaspoon margarine
6   ounces 1 percent milk
SNACK:
½ cup frozen yogurt
Total Calories: 1,480   Total Fat: 26 percent (38 grams)

Sample Low-Fat Menu for an Elementary School–Age Child
BREAKFAST:
4   ounces orange juice
1   cup oatmeal with raisins
8   ounces 1 percent milk
LUNCH:
½   tuna fish sandwich
1   ounce tuna packed in water (1 gram fat compared to 13
     grams in oil-packed tuna)
1   tablespoon fat-free mayonnaise (0 grams fat compared to
     11 grams in regular mayonnaise)
½   cup grapes
4   ounces low-fat yogurt
8   ounces 2 percent milk (school)
SNACK:
2   squares graham crackers
1   tablespoon peanut butter
4   ounces apple juice
DINNER:
3   ounces barbecued chicken (skinless breast) (4 grams of
     fat compared to 12 grams in fried chicken with skin on)
½   cup green beans

½   cup rice with 1 teaspoon margarine
8   ounces 1 percent milk
SNACK:
½   cup strawberry ice cream
Total Calories: 1,605   Total Fat: 25 percent (45 grams)

Sample Low-Fat Menu for an Adolescent
BREAKFAST:
8   ounces orange juice
1 ½   cups cereal
8   ounces 1 percent milk
LUNCH:
turkey sandwich
3   ounces turkey breast
1   tablespoon fat-free mayonnaise
lettuce and tomato
whole wheat bread
1   apple
1   ounce pretzels
SNACK:
6   gingersnaps
8   ounces 1 percent milk
DINNER:
4   ounces pot roast
baked potato with 1 tablespoon margarine
tossed salad with 2 tablespoons fat-free salad dressing (0
grams fat compared to 15 grams in most regular salad
dressing)
1   slice French bread with 1 teaspoon margarine
8   ounces 1 percent milk
SNACK:
Fat-free yogurt (1 cup)
Total Calories: 2,270   Total Fat: 27 percent (68 grams)

Ways to Lower the Fat Content in Your Family's Diet

DAIRY PRODUCTS
• Substitute low-fat or fat-free alternatives. For example, use low-fat frozen yogurt in place of ice cream; 1 percent or skim milk in place of whole milk; low-fat cheeses such as part-skim mozzarella or ricotta cheese.

MEATS AND FISH
• Choose the extra-lean variety.
• Remove all visible fats, including skin.
• Broil, bake, or grill instead of frying.

"ADDED" FATS
• Substitute low-fat or fat-free mayonnaise and salad dressings.
• Limit the amount of butter, margarine, sour cream, or cream cheese used in cooking or at the table (try substituting corn oil or olive oil for butter when cooking).
• Substitute marinara-type sauces for cream-based.
• Limit your intake of salads prepared with fat when dining out (for example, tuna salad, pasta salads, egg salad, etc.).

SOUPS
• Serve tomato-based or broth-based soups in place of cream-based.

DESSERTS
• Substitute ice milk, sherbet, Italian ices, or frozen yogurt for ice cream.
• Limit nuts and chocolate.
• Choose cakes and pies with lower fat content—for example, angel food cake over pound cake; blueberry pie over banana cream pie, etc.

3

❖ ❖ ❖ ❖

"The Sugar High"

One of the most prevalent myths is that refined sugar—more specifically, candy and sweets—causes children to become hyperactive, overtalkative, distractable, and difficult to control. The line of thinking—and many parents and educators zealously hold to this—is that the child's small body is overwhelmed by the "rush" of sugar as it is absorbed into his or her system, causing an overabundance of energy and excitability, followed by exhaustion, crying, or tantrums.

The "sugar high," if it exists at all, is a very rare situation. Sugar is not "speed." If sugar gave a buzz, or rush of energy, it would cost a few hundred dollars a cube. In fact, the myth of sugar per se causing hyperactivity has been tested and exposed. In blinded studies, teachers left the classroom while their children were given a variety of snacks—candy, apples, carrots, juice, or cookies. Back in their classroom, the teachers (who were familiar with those children) were unable to discern who among them had had the candy.

Once the subjective component is out of it, the sugar high proves undetectable—and yet parents will still say with conviction, "But I know *my* child and I know she gets hyper after having too much sugar."

Why is this?

It could be that the children have been cautioned or criticized so often about becoming hyper from sugar that they act the part expected of them.

It could be that they are so conditioned to sweets and candies being highly controlled that they automatically counter it with overexcitement and generally disruptive behavior.

It could be that the children's excitable behavior is connected with something totally separate from food, but to the parent it appears to be the result of food. A grandparent or some other favorite relative is coming for a special visit. Invitations to the child's birthday party have been sent out; the child cannot wait for the streamers, the balloons, the presents, the guests. Halloween is next week, complete with costumes, staying up late, and all that free candy. Some children, as soon as school starts in September, begin to squirm just thinking about Santa and all those presents!

In short, children have a million happy reasons to get excited, and having candy is only one of them.

Another possibility for children acting hyper is that they need an outlet for tension and, by coincidence, that need is timed with eating something sugary. This often occurs in a transition time from one activity to another, for example, being picked up from school or an after-school program, coming home and having a candy bar or handful of cookies, and then running all over the house, acting like a maniac. That is not a sugar high. Some children coming out of supervised settings such as school or after-school programs are often in need of releasing energy, and do so regardless of what they eat. Other children come home, eat a candy bar, and start "beating up on" their siblings when they have not seen them all day—a typical way children release tension.

Whatever the situation, there are very few children who at

five o'clock or whenever they are picked up docilely walk into the house, have a cup of juice, and sit down quietly to read a book. And if they do have a glass of juice, they are having just as much sugar as they would in a piece of candy, a cookie, or a piece of chocolate—the only difference being that the sugar in orange juice is perceived as "good" because it comes from nature (any excitability after drinking it would be ignored) and the sugar in the candy bar is deemed "bad" because it is manufactured (excitability after a candy bar will automatically be interpreted as misbehavior as the result of a sugar high).

From a nutritional standpoint, the "natural" sugar that is found in raisins and other dried fruits, honey, beets, or corn syrup is no better or worse for the body than the refined sugar found in cotton candy. Moreover, from a dental perspective, sticky foods like caramel candy are probably cleared away from the teeth faster than a piece of fruit because the sugar in carbohydrates, including candy, breaks down more efficiently.

How the Body Handles Sugar in the Diet

Understanding how the body handles sugar can help put the sugar high myth to rest.

The body eventually uses every form of dietary sugar in the same way—either immediately, by the cells in the body using it to provide energy, or fuel, to carry out their particular functions, or later by being converted first to fat or starch and eventually used as fuel. The "sugar fuel" gives us, therefore, what we might call the energy to carry out daily activities, but the sense of feeling energized depends not only on having the actual fuel, but on our mood, on whether we are healthy or not, and many other factors. The body is very efficient at maintaining a level of sugar in the blood to meet our energy needs, and only rarely does this system fail. Prolonged starvation (more than a week for well-nourished, older children or adolescents) or diabetes are examples where the sugar in the blood is inadequate or cannot be used for energy.

Sugar is not converted to hormones or chemicals that actually regulate our activity, nor does consumption of different amounts or kinds of sugar increase or decrease activity levels. The body is very efficient at keeping just enough sugar in the blood to meet our needs—all the rest is stored. The sugar in our diets is handled the same way regardless of our age, size, or the time of day we eat. In fact, we could eat something every hour or every six hours and the sugars are handled in the same way, keeping blood sugar at a constant level. The body also has good warning systems or signals to tell us if the sugar levels in the blood are moving down—we might get a little light-headed or experience a feeling of hunger.

However, as with excessive amounts of anything in the diet, sugar in quantities that children do not normally eat may not be digested well and can cause certain symptoms—for example, the "toddler's diarrhea" we see in as many as one in five children in practice. This is a condition in which otherwise healthy, growing, happy youngsters have frequent loose stools without any signs of malnutrition. For some children, excessive amounts of fluids or large amounts of fruit juices—that is, a quart or more of juice a day—can cause this, where a mix of drinks including milk would eliminate it.

When sugar is treated no differently from any other element in a child's diet, the myth of the sugar high is revealed for what it is.

A baby's taste buds are geared to accept sweets right away in first foods—breast milk is sweet, fruit juices and pureed fruits are sweet. Throughout life, most people associate sweets with pleasurable occasions. Every culture has some sweet confection associated with its traditional feasts and celebrations. A pleasant association of sweets with happy times and social gatherings probably helps children relax more than it makes them overexcited—unless of course they have been conditioned to associate sweets and candy with guilty moments or overindulgence.

Hyperactivity and Sugar— The Roots of the Controversy

Hyperactivity, attention deficit disorder, attention deficit hyperactivity disorder—all refer to the child who has a very short attention span, impulsivity, and is notoriously hyperactive or hyperkinetic—that is, who moves constantly and is all over the place, thinks very impulsively, and is easily distractable. These children drive teachers crazy and, in some situations, drive parents crazy before they reach kindergarten. (The age of onset is earlier than school age. Boys are more commonly affected by hyperactivity than girls.)

The sugar high myth became embedded into our culture during the 1960s, a time when many children were being diagnosed with hyperactivity. Part of the reason for that was the development of a new, easily administered questionnaire that, when a certain score was obtained, led to a diagnosis of hyperactivity (true hyperactivity occurs in only about 3 percent of all American children). With that surge in research, as well as the availability and effectiveness of the stimulant drug, Ritalin, to treat hyperactivity, many pediatricians began screening for hyperactivity. Stimulant drugs increase attention span and help hyperactive children to focus on an activity.

However, while the questionnaire was useful, it was not perfect. It gave many positives—too many—with the result that children who may not have needed drugs were put on them. At the same time, some teachers who discovered that Ritalin helped certain children concentrate better in the classroom recommended that more of their students be sent to pediatricians to get the drug. As a result, certain groups of schools and pediatricians around this time put a high number of children on Ritalin—and a controversy erupted.

When it could not be proven that sugar was the cause of difficult behavior in children, the focus of studies shifted to food additives. However, no hyperactive child eating a diet within the scope of anything we've ever seen—and that could include a lot of M&M's—has ever had his or her hyperactivity explained by additives.

THE SENSIBLE APPROACH TO SWEETS

- Avoid putting an emotional value on candy and sweets— i.e., using them as payments or rewards, or part of a bribe.
- Avoid outlawing candy or other sugared foods. Allow them in reasonable amounts along with a variety of other foods.
- Use the "five-a-day" guideline (see page 120) to give fruits and vegetables priority as snacks, as an alternative to candy and sweets to stave off hunger.

4

• • • •

Vitamins and Minerals: The Myths Dispelled

Certain myths and misconceptions about vitamins and minerals can create confusion about what children need to eat; this chapter addresses some of them. Although essential for health and growth, vitamins and minerals should not be overemphasized in a child's diet.

Misconception:
A Diet That Does Not Meet
Full RDA Percentages Compromises Growth

Surveys show that most American children receive 40 to 80 percent of the recommended amounts of vitamins and nutrients, an amount that is just right for them. The recommended daily amounts are deliberately set at a high level. This is to overcompensate for variations in the rate at which nutrients are absorbed, which is different for everyone. The RDA serves as a kind of "maximum safe allowance" without putting anyone in danger from having too much of a nutrient. Serious illness aside, we have yet to see an otherwise healthy American child who, with access to an abundance and variety of foods, has a vitamin deficiency, or whose growth has been stunted due to lack of specific vitamins.

Misconception:
Children Need Vitamin Supplements to Make Up for Erratic Eating

Children, even picky eaters, do not need vitamin supplements if they are given access to a wide variety of nutritious foods. When averaged over a few days, their daily diet supplies all of their vitamin needs.

One demonstration of adequate nutrition in American children is that, on average, they have become taller, heavier, and bigger than they were a hundred years ago, a trend that continues. Even during periods of rapid growth, most children still get all the vitamins they need without vitamin supplements. As their appetite increases, it triggers them to eat larger quantities of food, and this includes the foods that supply nutrients.

In periods of rapid growth, such as during infancy, supplemental iron may be required, and your pediatrician or family physician can advise you about this.

Although we do not recommend giving a pill unless it is necessary, parents who insist on giving their child a vitamin pill every day are doing no harm, provided their child takes it willingly. However, if the child needs to be coerced into taking it, then it is definitely better for the parent to stop making an issue of it. When a varied diet is offered, that child will thrive without vitamin pills.

Misconception:
Children Need Three Glasses of Milk
a Day to Obtain Adequate Calcium

We know of one mother who insists on three glasses of milk a day for her nine-year-old, soccer-playing son. She is sure that if he does not drink his quota of milk, he will not get enough calcium and his bones will be weak, putting him at risk during sports. However, this is not a well-founded concern. We have not seen any children who have fractured a bone for lack of drinking a "milk quota." Calcium is important to permit the bones to grow and remain strong. Its place in a child's diet for the mineralization of growing bones should not be confused with prevention of the condition called osteoporosis. Osteoporosis does not exist until the later years of life, and its causes are complex. The relationship of osteoporosis to the amount of calcium in the bones when we are children is unclear and still being investigated.

While those three glasses of milk will provide enough calcium for the day, that calcium can also be obtained in other foods (see list on page 116). Putting more calcium in the diet ("packing the bones") has not been shown to be advantageous for children over the long term; too much calcium may even cause some health problems in some children, such as kidney stones.

As for improving sports performance, calcium should be seen not as an issue for the athlete but rather as part of a balanced diet for a growing child, particularly during periods of rapid growth. A nine-year-old boy is not going through that kind of growth, and will not until he becomes an adolescent. At that time, with their natural increase in appetite, teenagers themselves will choose to eat more, including calcium-rich foods such as pizza, milk shakes, bagels with cream cheese, and any number of other foods that contain calcium—and other foods that give them the minerals and vitamins they need.

Misconception:
Vegetables Supply Children with Enough Iron

It all depends on the age of the child. In the middle years (ages three to eleven), iron requirements are low compared with those in infancy and adolescence, when growth is accelerated and the body's blood supply is rapidly increasing. Nursing infants get iron from breast milk or iron-supplemented formula, but adolescents need to pay special attention to their iron intake. Most of them are pounding away at sports (in athletes, the body's red blood cells turn over faster), and at the same time, they are growing rapidly. Adolescent girls who have started menstruating and adolescent vegetarians should also be aware of the need for iron in the diet.

Only about 1 percent of the iron from vegetables is absorbed into the body from the intestine, as compared with 10 to 12 percent of the iron from meat. Breast milk has the highest absorption rate of all—25 to 50 percent.

To be sure iron intake is sufficient, we recommend that young children through age five have their hematocrit (the ratio of the volume of red blood cells to the volume of whole blood) checked at least once by their pediatrician. This involves nothing more than a simple pinprick on the finger for the necessary blood work. In general, if your child's hematocrit is in the normal range—35 to 45 percent—and he or she is healthy and well functioning, there is no reason to be worried about iron. If it is low or you have a concern, then this should be discussed with your pediatrician.

Misconception:
It Can't Hurt to Load Up on
Vitamins and Minerals

In fact, it can be dangerous.

This is particularly true with the fat-soluble vitamins—A, D,

E, and K—which are stored in the body and can be toxic at high levels. Getting too much of these vitamins is rarely a problem, but it is possible to *make* them a problem, particularly if parents go on a megavitamin trip and decide to include their child on it, too.

In adults, toxicity problems with vitamin A can occur with doses of 20,000 to 25,000 international units (IU) a day for more than several months. In infants, this risk begins at anywhere from 4,000 to 25,000 international units for two months or more; in children and adolescents, it can occur with 40,000 IU and up, from six months to several years before symptoms occur. Problems that result from too much vitamin A can be serious, involving liver disease and pseudo-tumors—that is, symptoms of a brain tumor without having one.

Megadosing on vitamin D can be a problem, too. In the body, vitamin D is acted on by the liver and the kidney and turned into a hormone. As such, it circulates in the blood and stimulates the intestine to absorb calcium and phosphorus—the two principle minerals that account for the hardness of bone. Thus in normal amounts in an average diet (50 to 400 IU per day), vitamin D is beneficial as it increases the amount of calcium that is ultimately delivered to the bones. However, if you take too much vitamin D (more than 2,000 IU a day for months) and thereby increase the amount of calcium in the blood to beyond normal amounts, two major side effects can occur: arrhythmias in a regular beating heart and kidney stones.

Fortunately, the body has a wide tolerance for vitamin D by its "negative feedback route"—in the presence of too much vitamin D, the body stops forming the active hormone that promotes the uptake of calcium, and instead produces an inactive hormone that competes with the vitamin D, blocking calcium absorption. With an overdose of vitamin D, however, that negative feedback route can be overwhelmed and produce some serious problems, as mentioned above.

With vitamin C and all the B vitamins, there is no risk of an overdose because these vitamins are water soluble; excessive amounts pass out of the body in urine. However, too much vitamin C—that is, several grams of it—makes urine very acidic, and eventually stones may form in the kidney or in the bladder.

Misconception:
Increased Amounts of Potassium and Calcium Will Improve Sports Performance

It's much too simplistic to think that if you eat more of anything, the body will perform better. For an otherwise healthy child, loading up on vitamins or minerals will not improve a child's performance, physique, or immunity in any way.

We know of one situation where the coach of the high school wrestling team told a father that his son would have a stronger grip if he ate more bananas. The logic here was that if bananas contain potassium and muscles use potassium as part of their contractile process, then an increase in potassium would result in stronger muscles.

It did not seem to matter that the boy was at his ideal height and weight in relation to the growth charts; or that the gripping strength in his hands allowed him to be the best water-skiier at his camp; or that he was doing well on the wrestling team. The father followed the coach's advice and made sherbet banana shakes every night for his son, and got into fights with him about drinking them.

We were able to persuade this father off the potassium case, explaining that there is a variety of minerals needed for good muscle contraction—calcium, magnesium, and phosphorus as well as potassium.

Because it is essential to many functions, the body very efficiently accommodates safe amounts of potassium—absorbing what it needs from the intestine, holding a reserve in the cells of the body, and eliminating the rest. As most foods contain potassium, there is no point in going out of one's way to supply it; safe, adequate amounts are easily provided in the average American diet. Orange juice, for example, has more potassium than many other juices, but it does not make any difference if someone gets 400 milligrams of potassium or 200 milligrams from the juice because other foods will contribute to the 1,000 to 2,000 milligrams the body uses.

Under normal circumstances, too much potassium stimulates the body to get rid of it.

Trace Minerals There are a number of other minerals or metals that are necessary for proper functioning of the blood—selenium, chromium, iodine, fluoride, rubidium, zinc, and copper. These are called trace minerals, or metals, because the body needs such small quantities of them that they are readily supplied in trace amounts in almost anything that is eaten during the day, without the need to supplement them.

5

❖ ❖ ❖ ❖

Do Children
Need Fiber?

There is a place for fiber in a child's diet, but there are good reasons why a "bulky" diet should not be overemphasized for children.

Low-Fiber Diets Are Not a Risk for Children

Fiber is the indigestible, nonnutrient part of food that comes from plants—for example, the hulls from wheat or popcorn; the pulp or skins from apples and other fruits; seeds, rinds, and fibrous tissues from cooked or uncooked vegetables and beans. Fiber gives grains, fruits, vegetables, and legumes their structure at the same time that it provides roughage in the human diet.

While no one knows exactly how fiber in adequate amounts benefits humans (current theories center on its role in the prevention of cancer, diverticulitis, and heart disease), we do know that fiber contributes to digestion by encouraging involuntary muscle activity of the intestines so that the digestive tract functions normally, stools are soft and bulky, and bowel movements are regular.

Insufficient roughage in the diet, that is, a diet extremely low in fruits and vegetables that consists predominately of highly refined foods in which the fiber has been removed, such as white bread or white rice, can cause constipation and abnormal bowel patterns. Eventually a diet that is consistently lacking in fiber can, *in some adults,* cause other problems, such as diverticulitis, which is the inflammation of small sacs of intestine that protrude from the wall of the lower intestine. It is important to note that while such problems may be a concern for *some* (not all) adults whose diet is low in fiber—and diverticulitis occurs *in about one third of individuals over age forty-five and two thirds of those over sixty-five*—they are *not* a concern for children, even those children whose diet is low in fiber.

In addition, while problems from low-fiber diets are cumulative in adults, there is no proof or indication that they begin in childhood. Thus, while the eight-year-old whose diet is low in fiber may become constipated, this condition does not put him or her at any immediate risk for disease or illness and the parents should not even *think* of their child as being at risk. Instead, they should know that constipation can often be corrected by the introduction of fiber-rich foods into the overall diet.

Too Much Fiber May Interfere with Growth Needs

Adults who focus on the medical risks of a low-fiber diet (and who themselves may benefit from increased fiber in their diet) should think very carefully before increasing fiber in their child's diet.

The United States Department of Agriculture (USDA) and the National Cancer Institute, among others, have recommended that there be more fiber in the American diet; the Department of Health and Human Services has stated that less fat and more fiber would account for a substantial reduction in the number of cases of colon cancer in this country—in their estimate, 30 percent fewer cases and twenty thousand lives saved annually. While such statistics are hopeful and encouraging, growing children do not need a high concentration of fiber in their diet for two reasons:

1. *Too much fiber may interfere with the absorption of vitamins.* In the intestines, fiber acts like a sponge, binding to waste material and eliminating certain toxins in the intestines through stool movement. This is a potentially beneficial function because some of these toxins may be cancer causing. However, fiber also binds to vitamins, calcium, iron, and zinc, making them less "bioavailable," that is, less able to be absorbed through the intestine and into the bloodstream.

2. *Too much fiber fills a child up without providing nutrients.* High-fiber foods bulk up the diet and make a person feel full. This may be fine for adults cutting back on calories, but as fiber does not provide nutrients, large quantities of high-fiber foods may not give children the calories they need to grow. For example, unbuttered popcorn for a daily snack takes the place of roughly 500 to 1,000 calories of other, more nutritious foods that could have been eaten at that time. Popcorn remains a good snack, provided it is not the only snack food a child ever eats. Chocolate milk, cheese, bananas, carrots, peanuts, cereal packs, and other nutritious foods can be encouraged as snack variations.

While there is nothing wrong with white bread, and we cannot imagine a peanut butter and jelly sandwich on multigrain bread or dark rye, a diet in which white bread is the only food from the grain group is not going to contribute much fiber from that food group. Bran muffins, whole wheat bread and crackers, whole wheat pita bread, whole wheat flour, and brown rice are all good sources of fiber.

What We Recommend

Rather than concentrate on fiber per se, we recommend providing children with a variety of nutritious foods that include fiber—fresh fruits, vegetables, and foods made from unprocessed grain.

6

❖   ❖   ❖   ❖

Television, Children, and Obesity

There is a link between television and obesity, but television cannot be blamed for obesity, just as it cannot be blamed for lower intelligence scores or a passive personality.

The longer children watch television each day, the more likely they are to be obese—that is, the higher the *risk* of obesity. However, most children who watch television, even those watching more than two hours a day, are *not* obese. Television and obesity, then, may not have a cause-and-effect relationship, but rather an association. And some of the reasons people give for the association between the two is decreased activity, increased eating of snack food while watching television, and a sedentary life-style. As for determining which children *by nature* tend to be sedentary, again, television really cannot be factored into this as a cause. There were many sedentary and obese children before television, and even before radio.

In any case, we don't believe any of this is the way to look at the problem. The real issue for children is, for a particular child, how does television fit into his or her life?

In our opinion, making this determination is far more valuable to the child's well-being than flatly outlawing television or blaming it for problems.

To assess your individual situation, consider the following.

How Much Television Does Your Child Watch?

As recommended by the American Academy of Pediatrics, the guideline for television-viewing time for children is two hours a day. (In reality, many children watch much more than that, but so do many adults.) Much depends on how television time is used, relating to the children's stage of development. For example:

- Allowing an hour of *Barney & Friends* or *Sesame Street* for a young child while his or her mother tackles a few household chores or takes a break to read the newspaper is in a different category than using the television as an all-afternoon baby-sitter.
- For a tired, high-achieving elementary school student, a television break watching cartoons after school may help him or her relax. If that child has friends, plays outdoors, does well in school, and keeps up with his or her homework, we believe there is nothing wrong with allowing television shows, video games, or a rented movie after the child's homework is done in the afternoon.
- For the adolescent, turning off the fourth quarter of a football game or not permitting a late-night mystery because it exceeds the two-hour guideline would fly in the face of the adolescent's emerging autonomy (and hardly makes sense since soon that adolescent will be a college freshman making his or her own choices about what television to watch and what food to keep in the dorm refrigerator).

Does Television Time
Limit Reading or Homework Time?

You must be the judge of your child's individual situation and whether television cuts into reading time or schoolwork. There is no documented proof that television hampers intellectual development or learning. In fact, the National Assessment of Educational Progress, a government-financed study that has been tracking the progress of reading, writing, mathematics, and science skills among children, reports student achievement to be at about the same level in 1990 as it was in 1970—despite the fact that television watching among children ages nine, thirteen, and seventeen has steadily increased between those years.

Does Watching Television or
Playing Video Games Limit Time for
Social Life and Physical Activities?

There may be some merit in turning off the television set if TV holds a normally sedentary child back from joining with friends in outdoor activities, or encourages that child to eat when he or she is not hungry, but for most children in our culture (especially those who feel socially awkward or shy), television can help make them feel they are part of the group at school—by rehashing Super Mario's feats and adventures or retelling jokes from the last episode of the most popular sitcom.

If television gives the child something enjoyable to talk about with his or her friends, which in turn contributes to the child's happiness, seeing the show or playing the video game is far more valuable than having the parent outlaw it.

Do You Watch Television Together?

Watching television with your child—commenting on what you see on the screen—is an educational and entertaining process in itself. Not only does it give parents the chance to watch the popular reruns of the silly shows you spent hours watching as a child, but with parental guidance and editorial comment, it can also help the child learn to separate fantasy from reality, discern hyperbole, and recognize the sales pitch—for example, with product advertising that falsely promises a thinner, more becoming appearance and new popularity.

Watching the ads together provides a good opportunity for conveying the balanced nutritional message. Of course the information you give the child must be grounded in fact and not in myth. Telling him or her to "turn off the TV because it's advertising sugar and you know what sugar does to you," is only perpetuating the myth that sugar causes hyperactivity, as discussed in Chapter 3.

On the other hand, you can point out that despite what the candy ad says about vitamin C being added, candy is candy and still does not supply the variety of nutrients that come from other foods. While candy is fine for a treat, a variety of foods is important. That's the balanced nutritional message.

A Final Note:
The Place of Television in the Family

Television does create controversy; there are many questions about how it fits into family life that go beyond the scope of this book. For example, should violence and crime be treated as family entertainment? Do television shows and advertisements foster stereotypes or cast a harmful influence on children?

The answers to these and other important questions come down to personal opinions within individual families—well worth thinking about, discussing, and resolving within that individual context, particularly where there are young children living at home.

7

◆ ◆ ◆ ◆

Making Sense
of What You
Read and Hear

"Iron may increase the risk of heart attacks."
"Calcium may reduce the chance of future heart attacks."
"Breast milk is tied to higher intelligence scores."
"Fish oil saves lives."
"Contains No Tropical Oils"

Stop and think before shaping the family diet around what you read and hear.

To attract consumers, advertisers often exaggerate the link between nutrition and good health in their headlines and selling copy. While it is tempting to believe that certain foods can help prevent disease or prolong life, or that other foods can put one's health at risk, these are usually just theories. As many of the myths and conflicts over food choices originate from carefully crafted interpretations, this chapter presents guidelines for processing nutritional information accurately—in the media, in advertising, and on food labels.

Gleaning Real News from Hype

When the headlines on a food issue catch your attention, use these tips for putting them into perspective.

DO NOT CONFUSE INTERPRETATIONS WITH ORIGINAL DATA.

When data and study methods are interpreted for the reader, journalists and other writers can skew their interpretation of the facts to any degree they want. A topic can be presented as the new lifesaving treatment of the year or it can undeservedly be given a negative spin in order to catch the reader's attention.

A report last year linking chocolate to the prevention of cavities was a notable example of how data is manipulated to catch attention—and ends up causing confusion. The claim was presented in newsletter format to dentists, many of whom did not realize that the newsletter had been funded by the Mars Candy Company. In fact, the objective of the study, which was conducted by an oral biologist, Dr. Lawrence Wolinsky, an associate professor at the University of California at Los Angeles, was distorted in the newsletter. Far from encouraging the sales and consumption of chocolate, the objective of his study had been to isolate plaque-inhibiting tannins in cocoa and other foods so they might be used as additives in toothpaste and mouthwash. "Any gains you might get from the cocoa in chocolate would be more than offset by ingredients like sugar," Dr. Wolinsky said, when interviewed by *The New York Times.*

Negative interpretations were aptly demonstrated in an article that appeared in a special issue of *Newsweek* magazine in June 1991 entitled "What's in a Lunch?" reporting on school foods and the preference many school-age children show for fast-food choices at lunch. It painted an overall picture of children's health that would lead many parents to despair. For example, it stated, ". . . studies indicate that American children take in far too much fat and cholesterol for good health." This is an extreme statement. The most recent survey from the U.S. Food and Nutrition Service shows that children on the average eat 35 percent of their calories from fat, and have less than 300 milligrams of cholesterol per day. Those amounts are very close to the current recommendations by most major health organizations, including the American Academy of Pediatrics and the American Heart Association. The fact that 25 percent of children have cholesterol levels above 170 does not imply that 25 percent of children have *extremely* high cholesterol levels. In fact, extremely high cholesterol would be values greater than 213, and even with those high levels of cholesterol, fewer than half would have levels or risk factors serious enough to require specific intervention to reduce the risk of heart disease.

In the same article, the statement that "many children with high cholesterol show the first signs of heart disease" grossly overstates the findings. It takes approximately 60 percent occlusion, or obstruction, of the coronary arteries before an individual shows signs of heart disease. Autopsy studies in children dying from unrelated causes show that on the average, they have .1 percent occlusion. Furthermore, adult individuals with cholesterol values of 240 will reach this critical occlusion (60 percent) between the ages of sixty and seventy years, showing that the process is very slow and probably of no significance to children, adolescents, and young adults. The fact that these accumulations of cholesterol may be precursors is important to recognize, but it certainly does not signify that the arteries are clogged or that cholesterol has any impact for a given meal, in any week, month, or year.

To describe the number of obese children as increasing by more than 50 percent in the last twenty years, as is done in the same article, is also to overstate the data. The prevalence of *extreme* obesity has risen from approximately 17 to 25 percent in the last twenty years, but it does not follow that *most* American children are obese, or that 50 percent more American children today are obese than twenty years ago. Concerns about declining fitness and obesity in children are valid ones for our population as a whole, and yet reasonable solutions to them can only be found within the context of each individual family.

SCAN THE ARTICLE OR STORY FOR QUALIFIERS AS YOU READ.

Once again, headlines and sweeping statements are what sell. Look for qualifiers—words such as "may" or "could"—and details that may limit the bold claims. In that "Fish Oil Saves Lives" headline, for example, do not be surprised to discover a final sentence in the article explaining that the findings were based on a study of mice in Bolivia above three thousand feet. (In the meantime, it should also be noted that too much fish oil can cause liver damage.)

Whatever the claim, final proof that certain foods benefit the diet takes a long time.

RECOGNIZE THAT STATISTICAL OR RESEARCH SIGNIFICANCE IS DIFFERENT FROM CLINICAL SIGNIFICANCE.

There is a confusion in people's minds about what is statistically significant and what's physiologically or clinically significant—in other words, what relates to the health of the individual. This confusion occurs not only with lay readers but also with physicians and scientific readers.

An example of statistical versus clinical significance is the news feature describing a study about how calcium lowered blood pressure in children. In the study cited, however, only systolic blood pressure was measured, not diastolic, and the claim was based on seeing systolic blood pressure lowered 2 millimeters. What this means is that a child whose blood pressure would normally be 80 or 90 over 50, might be 78 over 50—a trivial difference! The commonly used blood pressure—measuring devices available to doctors cannot reliably measure that difference, and even if they did, a child's blood pressure normally varies by more than that when measured at different times. For example, if it were measured five times in a day, there could be a ten- or twenty-point variation between each measurement. In the blood pressure and calcium study there may have been a small statistical difference in blood pressure among children (78 versus 83), but clinically, that difference would be too small to have any significance to health.

KEEP IN MIND THAT NO MATTER WHAT YOU HEAR, DIET IN CHILDHOOD CANNOT BE LINKED TO LONGEVITY.

Adults often apply diet theories to children thinking it will protect them from future health problems. However, a single study that examines the effect of a particular nutrient on one parameter such as blood pressure, even over a period of a year, gives no information about the importance of that nutrient later in life.

Studies on health prevention and nutrition are extremely new and have yet to be followed through adolescence and adult life—that will take another thirty years. Thus, when children are studied—for example, when blood pressures are compared—it is very hard to compare two groups exactly, taking into account family histories, genetics, life-style, and personality types. As things stand, we do not know whether what happens at age three or age five has any meaning at age ten, fifteen, or forty, whereas fighting over what *not* to eat is probably going to raise everyone's blood pressure!

The same approach applies to lowering cholesterol and saturated fat in a child's diet: It has yet to be proven that eating a diet lower in fat and cholesterol when you are ten influences whether you develop a heart problem at age fifty-five, or even that it has any influence on what the child chooses to eat at age twenty or thirty. Young children usually go on to eat entirely different foods as adolescents, young adults, or parents. People make changes in their lives that researchers have no control over or knowledge about. As there is rarely money enough to fund long-term studies that would document those changes, it can never be absolutely clear that diet is the link with longevity, or with cardiac disease.

Therefore, whether through published data, efforts to revise food labels, or any other factor, within our culture right now it would be impossible to design a diet for any healthy child that would guarantee him or her increased longevity. While there is a consensus that lowering fat from very high to more moderate levels is a good idea, variations in genes, culture, and environment make exact dietary correlations with health impossible. Not only are these multiple factors inseparable but in combination they reveal a diversity of results. For example, while populations on low-fat, high-fiber diets appear to have a lower prevalence of heart-related deaths, apparently so do certain populations that use olive oil, drink red wine, or eat Brie. This is shown in countries such as France, Spain, and Greece, where people traditionally take in 40 percent of their calories from fat (much of it saturated fat) and yet do not die of heart attacks any more frequently than Americans do. If anything, they have fewer heart problems.

In Japan, on the other hand, the incidence of coronary heart disease has risen dramatically with the increase of fat and cholesterol in the diet over the last twenty-five years—this in addition to mounting pressures on Japanese society in terms of high-powered corporate life-style, crowding, and technological changes.

The Inuit tribe in Alaska has an extremely high-fat diet—50 to 60 percent fat—and a very low prevalence of heart disease. Clearly the presence of fat in their diet is for survival—and proof of why fat is so readily stored by humans. Most of us no longer depend on fat for survival against the elements, of course, making the storage capabilities of fat a liability for many of us, rather than a plus. Some people are not nearly as efficient at ridding their body of excess cholesterol as they are at storing it, or at protecting their arteries from the damage that can occur as cholesterol plaques develop.

All of the studies relating long-term diet to health are really too new to affect how and what we eat. We develop our eating habits over a hundred years or more, and it may not be the wisest thing to try to change them in a year's time or to try to change them month by month as little bits of new information leak out. It takes a long time for practical applications to become clear. In the meantime, we can use the information we have about the benefits of lowering fat—at the same time acknowledging that nobody is absolutely convinced of those benefits. All fats are not created equal, and there are even differences among saturated fats.

Interpreting Selling Copy

Certain words and phrases are used by advertisers to attract customers at the same time that they increase prices—for example, *organic, all natural,* or *cholesterol-free.*

If you do choose to buy products with these claims, do so with the knowledge that advertising and selling copy help shape their appeal. Selling copy—that is, claims that certain products are healthier than others—does not necessarily mean that other foods in similar categories are "bad" or unhealthy.

Here are some commonly used terms that are used as selling copy, and how we would interpret them.

"NO ADDITIVES, NO PRESERVATIVES"

Additives Additives include thickeners, stabilizers, and food dyes. Guar gum and xanthan gum, for example, are used both as thickeners and stabilizers. Guar gum is made from the guar plant; xanthan gum is made from corn syrup.

As part of a well-balanced, varied diet, there are no demonstrated health risks from the food dyes and additives in American foods today, and we have yet to see a patient for whom a food additive caused a serious health problem. (See Chapter 1 for a more detailed discussion.)

There is a difference between an allergic reaction and a chemical reaction. Although some people who have allergies are sensitive to certain food additives and react to them as to rugs or cat fur—for example, with itching, sniffles, or wheezing—they represent about 1 percent of the population and can thus be considered the exception.

As for chemical reactions, a common additive that can cause a chemical reaction is monosodium glutamate (MSG), used as a flavor enhancer. In a small number of people (about one to four in every one hundred) reactive symptoms range from a headache or tightening in the throat to chest pains or muscle aches. Although only a few people exhibit a reaction to MSG, to boost sales restaurants and food producers will advertise their food as containing "No MSG."

Preservatives Ascorbic acid, citrates, nitrites, BHT, etc.—these are all common preservatives found in preserved meats and in other foods, added to prevent spoilage, fungi, and molds that, if they occurred, would make a great number of people very sick.

Not only are the preservatives used safe (see Chapter 1 for more about the safety of preservatives) but the potential health risks of *not* putting them into foods is so great that, in our view, preservatives should be considered a boon to the population.

Food Substitutes An increasing number of "food substitutes" are becoming available, for example, the protein-based fat substitute Simplesse. Simplesse is egg white that has been finely mixed, or emulsified, into very small particles and when tasted duplicates the texture or consistency of fat. The drawback to Simplesse is that in cooking, instead of melting like butter in a frying pan, it fries like an egg.

Because the idea of a food substitute is new, for some people it raises immediate suspicion, and yet replacements for certain elements in the American diet, such as fat, are not such a bad idea. Food substitutes also include aspartame and saccharin, both of which have been rigidly tested to pass government safety standards for use in foods (see Chapter 1 for more on testing).

"ALL NATURAL"

The ad shows a baby in a cloth diaper, holding a shovel, standing in a garden; the copy boasts the creation of a baby food as natural as the baby—organic ingredients; grown without pesticides; never any added sugar; no cornstarch; no modified tapioca; never from concentrate.

The truth is it is impossible for most of us to understand the difference between what's natural and what is not—and whether "natural," raw, unbleached, and minimum processing are any better for humans than refined, bleached, and processed. "All natural" granola and granola snacks are a good example of what sound very healthy but in fact are very high in calories and in fat—they usually contain coconut and/or nuts. Moreover, if you look at the recommended serving size of some of those delicious, all-natural cereals, you see it is less than a half a cup—far less than most people pour into a bowl for breakfast.

All natural implies that if a food grows on a tree or a bush or comes directly out of the earth, then it is better, purer, or more nutritious than a food that has been processed in some way.

This is not always the case.

In 1993, there was an outbreak in the East of the same

bacterial germ that caused many people out West to become very sick when they ate tainted meat in certain fast-food restaurants. In the East, the source of the bacteria was traced to apple juice produced at a small apple cider mill. Some of the apples had been taken from the ground, where they most likely picked up bacteria from animal feces and other sources, and then were pressed for juice without first being washed, resulting in a few cases where people got sick with diarrhea after drinking it. This may be the exception rather than the rule, but parents who buy locally pressed cider may want to inquire if the apples were washed before pressing. However, while we are all in favor of fresh foods as part of a balanced diet—for example, vine-ripened tomatoes and vegetables picked right from the garden—it is one example of how the "pure, natural" route is not always superior to the supermarket route, and why you must be absolutely sure of the quality and preparation of the food you buy, including apple juice.

Another example of "all natural" not always being safe involves the danger of giving raw honey to babies. Fortunately, the FDA no longer permits the use of raw honey in infant foods—you may have seen cautions against it in your pediatrician's office—because although "raw honey" may sound better than a teaspoon of refined sugar and there's nothing wrong with it per se, it's much more dangerous to a baby because it can easily be contaminated with spores from botulinum and these spores can cause botulism in susceptible infants under one year of age. Many fresh, uncooked fruits and vegetables— lettuce, for example—can also carry botulinum spores, but babies, who are far more susceptible to botulism than anyone else and will outgrow that susceptibility, don't ordinarily eat lettuce or raw fruits or vegetables.

However, this is one good example of why "prepared" or "processed" baby foods are beneficial because naturally occurring risks have been eliminated, whereas uncooked or home-canned foods, even finely chopped, may put babies at more risk. The bottom line here is that a baby food from a big industrial company is no less natural or healthy than one that is "organically grown," and is probably less expensive.

"NO ARTIFICIAL INGREDIENTS"

Since all of us want to be as healthy as possible, advertising something as "natural" implies purity and health. In contrast, touting the idea of there being no "artificial" ingredients gives the latter a negative association. It is important to think about the goal of advertising—that is, to sell a product, not necessarily to promote health. As for the safety of "artificial ingredients," these are carefully monitored (see Chapter 1).

"NO PESTICIDES"

Pesticides are an environmental and political issue for many people, but in terms of food and food safety, they protect large food crops from being destroyed by bugs and insects—and even more important, stop the spread of bacteria that can cause enteritis, diarrhea, vomiting, and other symptoms. Washing vegetables and fruits before using them eliminates potential health problems (see Chapter 1).

"CHOLESTEROL-FREE"

Look for saturated fat content first, not whether the product is cholesterol-free. This phrase implies that dietary cholesterol is bad for everyone. However, dietary cholesterol may not be bad for you, and it certainly is not "bad" for a child. The recommendation that everyone over age two should limit dietary cholesterol to approximately 300 milligrams a day is reasonable, and with the help of your doctor you can determine whether your child is a candidate for selective screening of blood cholesterol (for determining factors, see page 34).

"NOT FROM CONCENTRATE"

When used in selling copy, the term *concentrated* has a negative connotation, but in fact juices made from concentrate do not lack vitamins or contain any less vitamins than juices that are freshly squeezed.

In order to process large quantities of fruits and fruit juices effectively, water is removed from the fruit, the fruit is packaged, and the consumer adds the water back in. The process of concentrating juices does not make them "unnatural" or harmful in any way; rather it comes down to economics (fresh costs more) and to personal taste (some people prefer fresh squeezed).

"NO STARCH"

Cornstarch, which is made from dried corn or, as the Indians called it, maize, is 100 percent natural and used as a thickener. There is nothing wrong or harmful about it, nor is a product inferior if it contains some cornstarch or tapioca to help keep it on the spoon.

Starch, a carbohydrate, is part of many foods. The more starch *added* to a food, the more calories in the food. However, most babies will adjust their intake over the course of a day when the foods they are fed are richer in calories than usual. This is similar to what happens when a baby is fed and takes in more cereal at a feeding—the baby eats less fruit or drinks less milk to compensate.

Making Sense of Food Labels

Food labeling is a mandated process spearheaded by the FDA to eliminate the many false claims that appear on foods— claims that cannot be substantiated with regard to health. With the new food labels, for example, claims that American cheese "builds bones," and that low-sodium turkey "lowers the risk of high blood pressure" will be eliminated because they are untrue.

The main objective of detailing label information is to substantiate claims—not to further complicate food choices! In our opinion, it is counterproductive to the goals of this book for readers to become deeply involved with label information, for example, for parents to use a calculator to compare label recommendations for servings with every serving of food they give their child—apple juice this morning, chocolate milk this afternoon, and water at dinner—and so forth. It is too microscopic a process to become mired in details; people should not be forced into strange eating patterns because what they've been accustomed to eating isn't going to meet what they think are the best standards. A better approach to the new label information is to use it to help balance out food choices, allowing certain foods that may not fall within strict guidelines, such as cookies that have 40 percent fat instead of 30 percent, as long as they balance out with a variety of other foods—some low in fat, for example, some higher in fat.

The goal of this chapter has been to help parents think carefully about the accuracy of the information that influences

---

How to Read a Food Label

1. Ignore the advertising copy.
2. Next, look for the balance (percentages) of fat, carbohydrate, and protein.
3. Is it high in fat? Does it contain other important nutrients, i.e., minerals and vitamins? Is it too expensive for what it contains? Do you want to buy it anyway?
4. When you base your choice of a product on the information given on the label, use it as a guideline in balancing out other purchases for family consumption—that is, if one is high in fat or lacking essential nutrients, balance it with another that is low in fat or high in nutrition.

food choices, and that may unnecessarily lead to restricting certain foods for children. The question remains, Why are some adults so susceptible, so ready or eager to take information that has very weak roots to it and adapt it as a way of life with conviction that's strong enough to cause arguments at the dinner table?

Part of it is the impulse to turn to science and technology to resolve our problems, save us from our sins, answer all our questions; part of it is a fascination with sensationalism—the desire to believe what we hear; part of it is a very normal desire to do the absolute best for our children—to protect them and try to give them happy and healthy lives.

Interestingly, many parents who readily agree that food should be a fun part of family life; that meals are a time to socialize with their children; and that good peer relationships and an overall sense of happiness or self-esteem are more important for a child's contentment and enjoyment later in life than any food issue will still latch on to shaky nutritional information and use it with a special vigor as a way to control their children. If you ask them which is more important, fighting over having salt on food or a child's feeling that he or she can have some sense of autonomy and independence at age twelve or thirteen, many of them will say autonomy and independence is key. Yet at the dinner table that night, they'll still cling on to the latest news story or to past knowledge that they think they have about nutrition and really give their kid a hard time.

So then the question comes down to what in the parents' own adult development makes them so vulnerable to using information in a way that both distorts what they know about their own child, and what they know is reasonable.

This type of situation warrants thinking about other issues—for example, the forced readjustment of personal expectations at midlife and how it may influence the wish for control, as discussed in Chapter 13.

◆ ◆ ◆

The Basics

8

❖　❖　❖　❖

Your Child's Growth: Establishing the Long-Term View

Is my child getting enough of the food she needs to grow? Many parents ask themselves this question as they cope with their child's erratic eating habits—uninterested in food one day, ravenously hungry the next, or fixated on the same food day after day.

To check whether a child is getting enough nutrition, you can measure and weigh the child, and compare these numbers on a chart with other children his or her age (see page 85). For further reassurance, especially when a child is not eating as well as you think he or she should, an overview of the growth years can put your concerns into a new perspective.

Growth is a steady, long-term process marked by certain predictable changes that will affect a child's interest in food and his or her appetite. Relative to this long-term process, as outlined briefly in this chapter, there is no way you can accurately determine—and no need to worry about—a child's health or growth on the basis of one meal, one day, or one week. Nor can you predict early on what the child's full-grown appearance will be, because over the course of childhood he or she can change dramatically. For example, a plump infant might turn into a slender child, who turns into a plump adolescent, who eventually becomes a tall and muscular young man or woman.

Normal Growth Begins with Weight Loss

Normal growth actually begins with a short period of weight loss during the first week or so after birth, when a healthy, newborn baby loses up to 10 percent of his or her weight in excess water. This is one of the few times during infancy and childhood when a child can be expected to lose weight. A seven-and-a-half-pound baby may drop down to seven pounds; a nine-pounder might weigh in at eight pounds, four ounces after the first week.

The water loss in the days after birth is a healthy sign that the maturing kidneys are functioning efficiently—it has nothing to do with undernourishment. At about the eighth or ninth day, weight gain resumes at the rate of about half an ounce to one ounce a day.

American babies typically double their weight somewhere between the third and fourth month and they continue gaining weight at about one-half to one ounce a day until about the fourth to the sixth month, when the rate slows down to about half that. Baby Anne is a good example of this typical pattern of growth. She weighed eight pounds, two ounces at birth, lost ten ounces in the next seven days; weighed seventeen pounds at five months; eighteen pounds, two ounces at seven months, and by twelve months had increased her weight to twenty-one pounds, six ounces. (Note: We include ounces because that is common pediatric practice. An ounce here or there makes no difference in measuring the baby's progress.)

Interpreting the Growth Curves

The pediatrician will weigh and measure a baby regularly, plotting the information on a growth chart to compare where that baby is in relation to other babies the same age. This is standard procedure all through childhood.

Interpreting the curves is easy. Of a hundred youngsters who fall within a range of normal lengths and normal weights, about 3 to 5 percent would be very much heavier or taller than the others, and about 3 to 5 percent would be much shorter or thinner. A child who falls right in the middle of that range is growing along the fiftieth percentile. A child lower than that might be growing along the twenty-fifth percentile, and a child growing on a higher curve than that might be on the seventy-fifth percentile.

If your child were measured along with those hundred children and his or her measurement were plotted on a curve for the fiftieth percentile, he or she would be of average height.

If your child were in the tenth percentile, he or she would be at the bottom 10 percent—in other words, 90 percent of the children measured would be taller or heavier than yours, and 10 percent would be shorter or lighter than average in comparison with yours—but everyone in the group would still be normal. (Use the charts at the back of this book to keep a record of your child's progress.)

Growth Is Initially Unpredictable

While the growth curves show a wide range of what is normal, in the beginning of a child's life they are not always accurate. It takes time for a baby to settle down into his or her curve.

Many parents and even some physicians do not realize that babies can take up to two years or longer to fit into their natural growth slot.

Newborn Billy's case provides the example here. Billy's parents considered themselves an average couple in weight and height. Billy's father was five feet, eleven inches in height and a relatively thin man; Billy's mother was five feet, two inches tall and of average weight. They expected their newborn child to be absolutely average—like most of their friends' infants, about seven-and-a-half pounds at birth. However, after a tough labor, Billy arrived weighing ten pounds, seven ounces! The nurse commented that he'd play football for sure, and his grandmother wondered if he'd benefit from a "diet" some time soon—to slow him down.

Billy proved them all wrong. Over the course of a year, this "big bruiser" at birth settled down into a growth pattern and by age one was slightly below the national average—but totally normal and consistent with his family heritage. By age seven, Billy was an average first-grader noted for his speed, not his size.

A Baby Is Just a Baby

As Billy proves, a baby at birth is often very chubby or very thin, and on a high or low weight percentile, and over the course of six to eight months may in fact drop or add several percentiles and then begin growing along his or her true percentile. Genetic traits are slow to emerge. In the meantime, there's no sense in worrying about every half pound or inch within a given normal range.

A fat or big baby is not automatically going to be a fat eight-year-old or ten-year-old—or even a fat adult. *A baby is just a baby* and, as demonstrated in several studies (see page 148), there is no reason for parents to be overly concerned about their baby's size or shape, or whether that baby is tall or short, thin or fat—*nor should they alter their baby's diet in any way,* as Billy's grandmother had considered, to try to meet expectations (see also page 202).

NAME _Billy's chart_

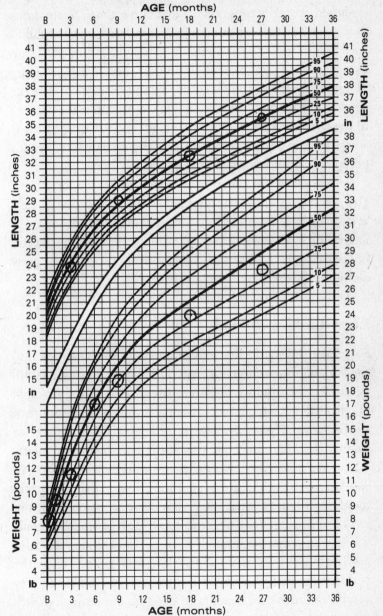

BOYS: Birth to 36 months
Physical Growth / NCHS Percentiles

The Gene Factor

Once growth has settled onto a curve for the individual child, it should normally progress on that curve. Small fluctuations at various intervals are not going to interfere with your child's final height potential as an adult. While the family physician or pediatrician pays close attention to where a baby is going along in percentiles, Billy's case is a good example of how the pattern of growth must also be looked at within the context of the family stature. Along with height and weight, *genetics* is a key factor in deciding what's normal for an individual, what's acceptable from a medical standpoint.

Billy began life at the ninety-seventh percentile for growth (length and weight); if he'd remained on that percentile, he'd eventually have been six feet, four inches tall at age eighteen and would have towered over his parents. However, by the end of the first year, he'd settled down several percentiles to grow along the fifteenth or twentieth percentile.

Every Child Is Special

Some time during the first and second year, a baby settles onto the length growth curve that will probably be his or hers until adulthood. Acceptance by some parents of where their child finally settles down on the curve may involve a compromise of expectations. They may have hoped for a taller, longer, or thinner child than the child they see before them, particularly if they are not happy about their own height or weight. (Of course, most parents are so enthralled with their offspring they forget about what they may have envisioned before birth.) However, if any of these issues emerge, and especially if they cause disappointment or concern, it is important to resolve them right away—by seeking reassurance from the pediatrician that everything is fine with the child, and by accepting the role of genetics in determining normal growth traits.

Jane was an adorable seven-year-old child whose mother brought her into the pediatrician's office with great concern about her size and stage of growth. For height, Jane was right at the fifth percentile—out of a hundred children, ninety-five of them were longer than she was. For weight, she was at the forty-fifth percentile. Her mother was five feet tall and about 130 pounds; her father was six feet, one inch.

If Jane's father had brought her in instead of her mother, and if we had never asked how tall his wife was, we too might have been concerned about Jane's growth and size. However, she was growing exactly like her mother—small, and with a little more body weight than average for her length—and would probably continue that pattern through her childhood and adolescence. Jane's weight might continue to be on the higher-than-average side for her age, but well within normal. For their weight, children who are in the heavier part of the curve do not necessarily or automatically end up being out of the normal range (obese) as adults.

When, if ever, should you be concerned about what the growth charts tell you? As noted, babies may actually drop or increase within two major percentiles before settling onto a curve toward the end of their first year—at their stage, that kind of movement would still be considered normal, although it would certainly be watched. In rare circumstances—for example, cases involving hormonal imbalances—if a baby's weight is very much out of proportion to length, it may be a clue to a medical problem, but weight and height that is out of proportion in the first few months is not an indication that such a problem exists.

Later than that, *any more than a twenty or thirty percentile change,* especially after the first eight months or so, would be a warning sign or clue that something has changed the youngster's eating pattern, activity, or behavior, and it should be checked.

Growth that appears to stop for six months or more or weight that changes dramatically in relation to length should be exam-

Summary:
How to Determine Normal Growth

• Plot height. Find your child's age at the bottom of the growth chart, put a ruler or straight edge on the chart at that point so that it goes from the bottom to the top of the chart. Find your child's weight (or height) along the side of the chart and draw a line straight across the chart to the age line. Where the two lines cross put a point. This point will lie on or between two of the heavy curves on the chart and represents your child's height/weight percentile.

• Plot weight.

• Check to see that percentiles are within normal range. (major percentile curves)

• Add genetic considerations.

• Any concerns, see your pediatrician.

ined for possible medical problems that may be affecting growth.

Jean, for example, has consistently grown along the thirtieth percentile for height and the thirty-fifth percentile for weight. At ten years of age, after her second winter of worsening tonsillitis, she dropped to the tenth percentile for weight while continuing at the thirtieth percentile for height. (The reason for this was loss of appetite—it hurts to swallow food when the throat is inflamed.)

The decision was made to remove her tonsils, and within a month after having them removed, her weight had increased back to her previous percentile pattern.

The First Year's Growth: Awesome

By the end of the first year, a baby will have grown at a rate never to be duplicated again in life. He or she will have tripled or even quadrupled in weight, increased ten to twelve inches in length (from an average length at birth of twenty inches) and, to accommodate the growing brain, increased head circumference by about eleven inches, from an average of fourteen inches at birth.

The energy needed to accomplish these feats will require large amounts of food on demand—of which approximately 50 percent of calories will be derived from fat. (For food requirements, see Chapter 2.)

A Slowdown in Growth from Age Two to Age Ten

Sometime between ages one and two, a child's rate of growth begins to slow down to a rate where it will largely remain until about age ten. This slowdown of growth is reflected in the child's diminished appetite—from a bottle or breast-feeding every three or four hours (day and night) to food three times a day with a few snacks in between. The decrease in the desire for food is completely normal—if the baby kept up that rate of food intake from the first year, he or she would weigh seventy-five pounds by age three—and yet it is quite typical for parents to worry when their toddler refuses food. Thus parents who are used to the high food demands of an infant may feel suddenly unsuccessful as their preschool child eats less or becomes fussy.

Billy's situation at this age is a good example. By the time Billy had reached two and a half years of age, his mother was concerned because he refused to eat almost everything she put before him. "RoboCop" spoons didn't help and in fact, most of Billy's food ended up on the floor or the wall. Billy's mom could not believe he could survive on the little bit he seemed to swallow, and she had run out of tricks and patience trying to get him to eat more. However, Billy's pediatrician observed an active, vigorous little boy whose length and weight placed him at the thirty-fifth percentile—the same percentile that he had been growing along since he was eight months of age. Billy's cheerful nature, normal development, and consistent gain in weight and length showed that, in spite of his "erratic" eating pattern, he was getting enough nutrition to keep his growth right on his normal growth curve—and he continued right along that way throughout his elementary school years, some days hungrier than others.

Accelerated Growth Resumes

When a child reaches puberty, growth accelerates at a rate that, while not as dramatic, is certainly as significant as the rate of growth in infancy. You can see this accelerated growth begin to occur on the growth charts, with girls around ages ten to eleven and with boys around twelve and thirteen. At this stage, it is not unusual to see a complete mismatch in the heights of the boys dancing with the girls at the junior high prom—the girls towering over their male partners by as much as a foot, and weighing a good twenty pounds more, when just a while before this, and all through their previous years, the girls and boys had had similar heights and weights.

The "growth spurt" that accounts for the changes in height and maturation has a different timetable for individual children. Some children approach their full adult height at twelve or thirteen; others do not begin to accelerate until later in their teen years. Often those who end up being the tallest children, if they enter puberty later than others, tend to be at "the middle of the pack" for a while as the children who mature earlier temporarily spurt ahead of them.

Throughout this awkward time, boys and girls are consistently interested in their linear growth. Very few of them want to end up being very short, yet of course there's nothing wrong with that. A medical exam is not necessary for charting growth; just drawing a line on a closet door with a ruler perpendicular to the top of the head and watching the marks climb up toward the ceiling is enough. The Tanner Growth

Velocity Curves (see page 271) are especially helpful in reassuring teenagers of their progress, whether they are "early" or "late bloomers." Instead of measuring the actual height at a given age, these charts measure an individual's progress by how much he or she has grown in one year—for example, three inches, age ten; four inches, age eleven; five inches, age twelve. You can make a curve out of those points and see much more readily than on a standard growth curve whether the youngster is going through a growth spurt over a period of time.

Most adolescent girls want to be thin. Most adolescent boys want to be muscular. As Dr. David B. Herzog, pediatrician and child psychiatrist on staff at Massachusetts General Hospital, has pointed out, when you interview teenage boys, 30 percent of them will say they want to be bigger and bulkier, and when you interview the same number of girls, all of them will probably say they want to be thinner. Parents need to recognize that those two differences exist during adolescence, and should try to work with the individual child to help him or her achieve body and weight goals within reasonable limits (see page 190).

In many girls, hormonal activity that triggers the onset of menstruation typically brings a weight gain. There is a theory that for girls to begin their menses, they have to have a certain amount of body fat. This is probably *not* true, at least for girls who are in the middle range of percentiles, but the observation has been made repeatedly that the onset of menses in girls at far extremes (thin or obese) is influenced by the presence, or lack of, body fat. Specifically, girls who experience sudden weight loss and are extremely thin in their preadolescent years will not develop their menses at the same time as their peers, while truly obese young girls tend to have earlier menses.

Dr. Rose Frisch, an epidemiologist at the Harvard School of Public Health, related these findings in a report published in *Science* magazine in 1974—specifically, that a certain amount of body fat is necessary in some way to regulate the hormonal changes around puberty bringing about the onset of menstrual cycles. However, it is important to note that *these findings involve girls who are at far extremes in terms of their body fat and weight*. Obviously, the onset of menstruation is influenced by genes and other factors as well, and for girls of average weight, will be determined by a combination of these factors.

Watching for Adolescent Growth

Between ages twelve and sixteen, parents can discreetly look for signs that their child is beginning to mature. In girls between ages ten and twelve, body changes include breast development, underarm and pubic hair, body odor, fat redistribution to thighs, and the onset of menstruation. In boys between ages twelve and fourteen, they include a deepening voice; facial, underarm, and pubic hair; body odor; and increased muscle mass. If your child suddenly needs new shoes twice a year or longer pants twice a year, that's a clear indication that his or her growth has accelerated.

When should a parent be concerned about adolescent growth? While rare, if there is no indication of any of the changes described above in your child by age sixteen, or if certain changes such as very early breast development concern you, discuss them with your pediatrician.

In any case, it is a good idea for preteen boys and girls, from age ten on, to visit their pediatrician annually (it can be the annual visit for school or camp health forms), not only to check physical health and keep up with booster shots, but also to discuss personal concerns or questions about body changes and risky behaviors. Parents should encourage adolescents to speak freely with their doctor, who should be more than receptive to offering counsel.

While respecting a child's increasing need for privacy, a parent's sensitivity to adolescent behavior, moods, and attitudes is especially important during puberty and adolescence.

If a teenager (or any child, for that matter) is barely dragging him- or herself out of bed in the morning, coming home with poor grades, keeping aloof, falling asleep the minute he or she gets back from activities, it is possible that the teenager may not be getting enough food or sleep, or may be feeling stressed or depressed.

These are warning signs, not only for diet but for other aspects of a child's life that a parent can pick up on and help with—obviously, not waiting to discuss them with the pediatrician until the next routine visit if they cannot be resolved.

Growth in the Final Analysis

Neither growth curves nor genetics can predict exactly where a child ends up in height or weight as an adult. Culture and environment play a part throughout childhood in influencing a child's appearance, and yet in some cases it may not be until the young adult stage, when the child has moved out of the home and away from the family's established eating habits, before his or her individual weight is finally determined. Up until then, genetic traits can be masked by environmental determinants, primarily the family diet. This can happen when children are placed on overly restricted diets. It is also true in families in which parents are very overweight, since children of such parents also tend to be overweight. Yet often these children will fall into a more normal weight range once they

---

Highlights of the Growth Years: A Summary of What to Expect

Baby's First Year	Very Rapid Growth
Age 1 + to 2	Slowdown of Growth
Middle Years, 2 through 10	Slow, Steady Growth
Adolescence	Accelerated Growth in Puberty

are out on their own. There is no evidence demonstrating that weight reduction during childhood ultimately influences the child as an adult.

Parents who feel tension or pressure over their child's progress and development need to step back and look at what makes them susceptible to the idea that a child should grow a certain way. Does the pressure come from comparisons with other children in the neighborhood? Unrealistic standards and concerns of grandparents or peers? Cultural prejudices, such as the acceptability of tall men and thin women?

Parents who need confidence in withstanding these and other pressures will benefit from cultivating a more realistic sense of normality, accepting that there is no one standard or way of parenting and that throughout childhood, "normal" covers a wide spectrum of differences among happy, healthy children, whatever their stage of growth.

9

❖ ❖ ❖ ❖

Food for Growth

The Growth-Energy Connection: So Different from Adults

Children need food and the energy it provides to sustain their growth. They're not trying to maintain the steady number of pounds adults would love to see when they step on the scales, nor do they need to adjust their calorie intake to the slowdown in metabolism (the rate at which calories are used) that occurs in a middle-aged body.

In comparison with most adults, the energy expenditure by children is very high: The healthy adolescent schoolboy who plays soccer or ice hockey can burn 4,000 calories a day while his office-working parents may burn less than 2,000 calories.

Obviously, the child who burns high quantities of calories in physical activities needs many more calories in his or her diet than an adult or an inactive peer does in order to maintain optimum weight. But children are also using calories *just by growing* and their calorie requirements at different stages reflect this "cost for growth."

For comparison, look at what a healthy baby needs in calories *for growth alone* as compared to the needs of a child between ages two and eleven, and an adolescent between ages twelve and eighteen. Doubling their birth weight in the first four months and tripling it in the first year, babies typically consume an average of 50 to 60 calories per pound each day for growth, activity, and the energy needed to metabolize food—that's more than *three and a half times the calories per pound needed by a twenty-year-old.* Babies have small stomachs in proportion to their calorie needs; they need a rich concentration of calories and frequent feedings to sustain growth at such an accelerated rate. By the second year, the calorie needs (for everything) have slowed down to about 40 calories per pound and then to 25 to 35 calories thereafter to about age ten. As growth accelerates during puberty, the adolescent again needs about 30 to 40 calories per pound.

This energy cost for growth can be measured in percentages. For the baby, it represents a full 20 percent of total calorie requirements, whereas for the child it represents only 1 percent, and for the adolescent it picks up again to approximately 2 percent of caloric intake—not nearly as dramatic as for the baby, but double the cost for growth of the younger child.

Although we look at *total* calorie requirements in determining a child's optimum diet or food intake (see Chart II, page 110), these cost-for-growth comparisons are important as they show why there is a special need for foods that will provide concentrated nutrients and a high number of calories, or energy, during infancy and in adolescence, two predictable phases of rapid growth.

Different Foods
Have Different Energy Values

An easy way to look at the difference between low-energy foods (low in calories) and high-energy foods (high in calories) is to look at how much energy you get out of an apple or bowl of popcorn as compared to what you get out of a roast beef sandwich or a steak. Apples and popcorn are low-energy foods; they provide fiber and vitamins but you would have to eat about six apples to equal the calories, or energy, you get out of the roast beef sandwich.

Obviously, children who are in a fast-growth period do not need to follow a high-protein diet and have a roast beef sandwich for a snack every day or a steak every night, but how is the active teenage athlete who is burning 4,000 calories a day doing gymnastics or figure skating or ice hockey going to get 1,000 calories in a sitting to replace those calories?

That teenager needs to eat three full meals a day and snacks that provide a wide variety of high-protein, high-calorie foods. Foods such as popcorn or apples are a fine snack choice for everyone, including the teenager, but fiber fills you up without providing calories. High-fiber foods such as these are great for alleviating hunger, but for the athletic teenager who is going through a growth spurt, he or she would be doing so without consuming the calories needed to provide the energy to support his or her activity level and growth.

Our Basic Principle
for Supplying Nutritious Food

To ensure that a child receives the food he or she needs for growth is simple:

Make nutritious food available to your child at all times. In periods of rapid growth (under age two and during the adolescent growth spurt) increase the availability of high-energy (high-calorie) foods for snacks and meals.

It is up to the parent to provide a variety of foods that will supply energy and nutrients; as for quantities of food to be eaten, the child's appetite makes that determination (age-appropriate foods are detailed below).

The Place for Fat in a Child's Diet

This is also different than for adults, as fat is a concentrated source of energy.

From birth to age one, children consume a diet that supplies over 50 percent of its calories as fat—that's almost double the amount recommended for adults (25 to 30 percent).

At about age two, the requirement for fat decreases: Not only has the child's growth rate slowed down, requiring fewer concentrated calories, but by then nutrients are more easily obtained from a wide variety of foods.

After age two, as detailed below and shown in the sample menus, page 150, a varied diet should ideally include approximately 30 percent of its calories from fat (with less than 10 percent of those calories as saturated fat—the same as for healthy adults); 10 to 15 percent of calories from various sources of protein such as meat, poultry, fish, and dairy products; and 50 to 55 percent of its calories from cereals, grains, beans, and other complex carbohydrates—a balance that will continue supplying the essentials needed for growth throughout childhood and adolescence.

If you are worrying about fat or cholesterol in children under age two or, for that matter, about anything else in their diet, such as "fat versus protein" or "salt versus no salt," you need to step back and rethink your position. Virtually all health experts agree and emphasize that no attempt should be made to lower fat in the diet of infants and young children from birth to age two, but instead, the diet should be geared to maximize growth. Once again, fat, for babies most intensely, is an important food source for growth.

When seen in this light, clearly *almost all of the nutritional advice we follow for ourselves is irrelevant and potentially harmful when applied to babies and children under two,* and for 99 percent of all babies, parents should not be concerned about overfeeding, fat, or the fat content of their baby's food.

If you find yourself trying to apply any other dietary information or adult issues to children under age two, speak to your pediatrician, review the first part of this book (and keep reading further!) and realize that something is going on in your head that does not make nutritional sense.

Applications:
What Children Need to Eat

In Chapter 8, we outlined the stages of a child's growth. Here, we present specific foods for the three phases of childhood nutrition—from the baby's high-fat liquid diet and the introduction of first solid foods, to the varied foods that will make up a balanced diet for the older child.

THE HIGH-FAT LIQUID DIET: ALL AN INFANT NEEDS

For the first four to six months of life, we recommend an exclusively liquid diet of either breast milk or infant formula for babies, both of which are more than adequate as a complete food for a baby. Breast milk and infant formula have an equal value of fat (approximately 50 percent); both deliver in small volume the amount of energy-rich nutrition an infant needs for growth. Breast milk also contains cholesterol, which, for a baby, is essential for building cells in the body and brain. Infant formulas have minimal amounts of cholesterol, but this is not a problem or a drawback because the main source for cholesterol in the body is the liver, where it is manufactured. (Many people do not realize that all through life, only a small percentage of the cholesterol used by the body actually comes from food.)

Whole cow's milk isn't optimal for a baby (to age one year) because it is not digested well by the very young infant and contains too little iron, zinc, vitamin C, and vitamin E to support the baby's rapid growth and development. Cow's milk also may have too much protein, calcium, and phosphorus to help the baby's bones grow and develop optimally.

To Breast-Feed or Bottle-Feed? This question can pose a problem to mothers who, because of their peers, their cultural background, or some other factor, may feel judged as parents by the way they feed their babies. Parents should make a fully informed decision on whether to breast-feed or use formula. Information to help in making the decision can be obtained from reading, classes, the obstetrician, the family practitioner and the pediatrician. A prenatal visit with the pediatrician can be very useful in this regard. Babies can thrive with either method of feeding. Parents should recognize that during the second six months of life their breast-fed infant may be thinner than other infants who are being formula-fed. Parents should not view the thinner infant as less healthy and the fatter infant as healthier. The length of breast-fed and formula-fed infants is very similar.

The media is often no help to the woman who feels pressure in deciding how best to feed her baby. For example, in 1992 there were news reports on a study done in England, with headlines proclaiming that breast milk for premature babies is tied to higher intelligence scores. The implication was that breast-fed babies are smarter than formula-fed babies. Although that would be great if it were subsequently proven to be true, the report must be looked at with caution for several reasons. This study only dealt with small numbers of premature infants who may have had age-related neurological problems that were not taken into account. It was also hard to ignore that *twice* as many mothers had higher levels of income and education in the breast-feeding group, thus giving the breast-fed babies an environmental advantage over the formula-fed babies. The breast-fed babies were reported to test "eight points higher," but it was not specified what eight points higher on a range of tests meant—were they better with language, memory, calculation, abstract thinking? (In any case, eight points is a very marginal difference in measuring intelligence quotas.)

There is evidence that breast milk lessens the possibility or severity of infections because of immunities the baby receives in the milk. Although these benefits have been difficult to demonstrate in developed nations, such as the United States, where in general the water supply is clean and uncontaminated, recent studies have shown a lower incidence of ear infections and upper respiratory infections in breast-fed infants here and a markedly lower risk of lower respiratory infections, diarrhea, dehydration, and hospitalization for the exclusively breast-fed infant in developing countries. The mother who plans to bottle-feed her infant might consider breast-feeding her newborn for at least the first several weeks or so after birth, when there is a high concentration of protective factors in breast milk as well as highly concentrated nutrition.

What about attachment—or "bonding"? While one of the advantages proposed for breast-feeding includes the bonding between the mother and the infant, the correlation has never been proven as to whether a breast-fed baby is ultimately happier or has a better character or is more emotionally secure than a formula-fed baby. From a psychological viewpoint, the thought of people bonding has, in any case, always bothered us. Glue bonds. Geese and goslings bond, based on visual contact and following behavior in the first hours of life. Bonding, in these terms, suggests a chemical or neurological, locked-in process that, like epoxy, must be timed. We prefer to think that people attach. Clearly a formula-fed baby with a mother who loves her baby, holds her baby, and spends time with her baby is going to be as fine a human being as the breast-fed baby.

As maternity leaves for working mothers are relatively short, breast-feeding after 6–8 weeks may become more difficult. Mothers who wish to breast-feed, however, should be encouraged to continue doing so and should be provided with every possible support. This includes providing instructions on pumping the milk, storaging, transporting, and feeding of the milk while the mother is at work and the infant is at home or in a day-care setting.

Scheduling Food In the first few days after birth, most babies should be offered food "on demand" (that is, whenever their behavior or facial expression indicates hunger). Although crying and fussiness may be a clue that the infant is hungry, parents can usually learn to interpret hunger cues before the infant reaches the crying stage. Feeding the very young infant every 2–3 hours, or as often as they seem to need it and without restriction, leads to appropriately frequent nursing and in turn leads to development of a good milk supply in the nursing mother. If they continue to cry after being fed it is reasonable to offer a pacifier—particularly for the older infant since sucking provides comfort and this may be what they need (for more on pacifiers see pages 179–180). Whether an infant is fed on demand or on a schedule, parents should be flexible about offering food and recognize that the baby may want to fix or adjust his or her own schedule. With breast-fed babies, since sucking stimulates milk production and the release of milk from the breast, the length of time the baby is on the breast at a feeding is important—it should be a minimum of 10 minutes at each breast per feeding, starting each feeding with the breast last offered.

How to Tell if a Baby Is Getting Enough Food This is a real concern for many parents of new babies, especially newborns who are being breast-fed by mothers who are new to breast-feeding. Growth is the best indicator. Healthy, full-term infants should have no trouble digesting human milk or infant formula, as evidenced by their steady increases in length and weight.

At two to four weeks old, a formula-fed baby usually drinks about two to three ounces of formula per pound per day. That does not mean the baby has to finish every feeding, but at least you can watch to see how much food he or she is getting.

To check whether breast-fed babies are getting enough food, you can have them weighed at regular intervals at the pediatrician's office and you can go by what you see in the diaper. There should be frequent wet diapers (for the breast-fed infant at least six wet diapers per day in the first few weeks of life) and evidence of stool. (Different milks produce different stools; those produced by breast milk are usually seedy, yellow, and sporadic—they may occur with every feeding, or only every three or four days, but that is not a sign of a digestive problem.)

Sometimes breast-feeding skills present a problem—for example, a new mother may have considerable difficulty positioning the baby on the breast, or the milk does not seem to flow freely. In that case, seek out advice from an experienced friend or relative, or from a breast-feeding support group or specialist in "lactation counseling," whom you can find through your pediatrician's office or local hospital.

Fortunately, for both breast-fed or bottle-fed babies, there are several ways to tell if things are going well:

- *Watch the baby's behavior.* While first attempts by the baby to initiate feeding are typically somewhat weak, by the second day of life babies will generally become well established on the breast or on the bottle. Breast-feeding can, and in many cases should, be initiated within 30 minutes to 1 hour after birth. You want to see by their rhythmic sucking action that they are actually swallowing milk.
- *Check to see that the baby is having frequent stools and that the diaper is frequently wet.* A baby may be passing anywhere from three to seven stools a day, or after the first few weeks, as seldom as every four days, but those stools will not resemble those that result from solid foods. In a breast-fed baby, they may resemble something more like birdseed.
- *Call the pediatrician.* While parents should not be encouraged to weigh their baby day by day, they should not hesitate to call the pediatrician in particular for advice about breast-feeding and also if they have concerns about whether their

newborn baby is getting enough food. And by all means they should consult the pediatrician if the baby is (1) quieter and sleepier than a normal baby should be; (2) very irritable, or crying constantly; (3) less interactive even for a new baby; (4) passing very little urine; or (5) not gaining weight, or losing more that an ounce or so a day in the first week.

These are all warning signs that the baby may not be getting enough food, and they warrant advice and possibly an examination. Babies are fragile. Be persistent in getting through to the doctor with your concerns, and in making an appointment.

A Summary of Feeding in the First Four to Six Months Feed your baby breast milk or formula, on demand or on a schedule. If you have concerns, discuss them with your pediatrician or family practitioner who will also help you monitor your new infant's growth on the appropriate charts.

(For more on early interactions with a baby, turn to "The Newborn and the Postpartum Adjustment," page 173.)

THE TRANSITION TO SOLIDS

About halfway through the first year, babies begin to outgrow their liquid diet of human milk or formula, which, because of their increasing size, can no longer supply them with enough calories to support their rate of growth. For most infants, soft foods are introduced between four to six months—for both a bottle-fed and breast-fed baby. This second phase of childhood nutrition is a time of transition—from the infant diet of milk (although for the first four to six months, milk still supplies 100 percent of the baby's nutritional requirements) to soft foods, finger foods, and finally, with a full set of baby teeth, to family foods. During this phase of growth, babies move from being totally dependent on parents for food and feeding to feeding themselves, mastering the eating skills that will enable them to join the rest of the family and eat what everybody else eats.

Some parents want to start solids before six months because

they think the baby is hungry, is crying for more food, can never survive on a liquid diet, or needs solid food to sleep through the night. Usually this is not the case. For some infants, however, solids can be given earlier to help the baby gain weight if he or she is not gaining well. This sometimes happens when the baby is spitting up frequently. Thickening the milk with cereal sometimes reduces the spitting (or reflux) and also provides some extra calories. That can be seen on the growth curve and discussed with your pediatrician. Otherwise, before four to six months, you can rest assured that the baby is getting all the nutrition he or she needs from milk (breast milk or formula), and leave it at that.

If you still want to give solids earlier than six months, that's fine, but if you have ever tried feeding a three-month-old with a spoon, much less keeping the food in the baby's mouth, you will know it is quite difficult because of the baby's extrusion reflex—the tongue pushes things out of the mouth. This normal reflex in young infants disappears somewhere between the fourth and sixth month of life, right on schedule for introducing solid foods, when the tongue begins to move food toward the back of the throat, rather than push it out.

FIRST SOLID FOODS

For their introduction to solid foods, babies are usually propped up in an infant seat and by about a year to fourteen months, they are usually well established in a high chair in the kitchen, eating with the rest of the family, although not yet fully participating in the family foods. If not sitting up in the high chair to eat, the toddler is probably fighting to get out of it, generally uninterested in food and eager to get down on the floor, look around, fiddle with things, explore the world and, most important, master it. (See also "Baby to Toddler: The High Chair Adventure," page 181.)

So that allergies or food intolerance can be detected, babies are usually introduced to solid foods (pureed or strained) with one single-ingredient food at a time and one food group at a time—first, grains, then fruits and vegetables, and finally meats—one new food each week. (Infant rice cereal mixed with formula or breast milk represents a typical first food offered to the baby for one week before introducing another food.)

This systematic approach generally takes one month to one and a half months from starting one new food group to the next, with *foods that are thought to be allergenic, such as eggs, peanut butter, and fish, delayed until close to a year in age.*

(For more on allergies, see Chapter 18.)

At each feeding, small, baby-size servings of one to two teaspoons should be offered, increased gradually to portions of two to four tablespoons per feeding. A good rule of thumb for serving size of any food is one tablespoon for each year of age, up to age eight. Taking seconds is much more pleasant for the child than having a heaping mound of food placed in front of him or her; one-half cup of peas for a two-year-old may be three times what he really needs.

Once fruits and vegetables are established, include one good source of vitamin C and one good source of vitamin A in the baby's daily diet (see lists, page 116).

Up through the first year, formula or breast milk still provides most of the necessary daily calories a baby needs. Between six and eight months of age, as soon as they show an interest in holding it, babies can be encouraged to use a lidded cup. Introduce juices in the cup at about six months, and begin placing some of the infant's milk in a cup at seven to eight months. Use real juice (not fruit drink) with no added sugar and limit the amount to eight ounces a day so that the nutrients from formula or breast milk are not completely replaced by juice.

Iron and Infants While children get all the vitamins and minerals they need from the wide variety of foods in a well-balanced diet (see "Where They Get Their Vitamins," page 111), rapid growth in the first year requires extra attention to a baby's supply of iron so that iron deficiency or anemia will not result. Fortunately, while there is only a small amount of iron in breast milk it is sufficient and readily absorbed by the infant, and infant formulas are iron-supplemented. Cereals fortified with iron are another source for iron.

Infants drinking regular cow's milk before ten to twelve months (although this is not recommended) should have an iron supplement prescribed by the physician. (For more on iron, see below.)

Vitamin Supplements In nearly all cases involving healthy children, the choice of whether to give vitamin supplements or not comes down to parental preference. From a nutritional standpoint, babies and young children do not require supplemental vitamins if they are eating a variety of foods by the time they are nine or ten months of age.

The only notable exception to this involves the breast-fed dark-skinned infant who may need a supplement of vitamin D to ensure that he or she is making use of the minerals in the milk to produce strong bones. As the need for vitamin D varies from individual to individual, the pediatrician should make the determination of whether vitamin supplements are necessary.

By *eight to ten months of age,* the average baby will be eating a variety of foods from the fruit and vegetable group and from the bread and cereal group—but do not be upset if your idea of varied diet or healthy appetite does not match that of your child's. Children do not have to be force-fed at any given meal to meet their calorie requirement. Keep offering a variety of foods. As long as you make nutritious food available to them in reasonable portions and *you don't get caught up in battles over food,* children will normally eat what they need to keep growing appropriately on the curve.

Introduce textures to correspond with the baby's ability to chew, that is, as teeth come in. Mashed or chopped foods are suitable for "gumming," but with the appearance of incisors (front teeth), babies are usually ready for soft "finger foods"— cooked fruits and vegetables cut into small cubes, or pasta that can be picked up by small hands. Introduce meat and meat substitutes (poultry, fish, etc.) very finely ground and one variety at a time, again, waiting about six to seven days between each new food to be tried.

Foods to Avoid

Round, hard foods such as nuts, candy, gum, grapes, popcorn, raw carrots, raw green pepper, chunks of hard cheese or hot dogs may cause a baby to choke and should be avoided until the baby is at least age three.

By the end of the first year, most infants will have been introduced to a wide choice of pureed, chopped, and finger foods from the basic food groups of milk and dairy, grains, vegetables and fruits, and meats (see below). Around twelve months, babies can switch to drinking whole cow's milk. *(Low-fat milk products are not recommended until after age two.)*

From age one on, children are ready to begin consuming "real" foods, in child-sized portions and cut into pieces they can chew.

THE VARIED DIET

The third stage of childhood nutrition encompasses the years when children are old enough to manage adult food. Individual requirements for calories and food amounts vary among children, depending on their rate of growth and activity level. Generally speaking, however, Charts I and II show what all children need for good health and growth:

Chart I
WHAT CHILDREN NEED TO EAT
Recommended Dietary Allowances

For good health and growth, your children (older than one year of age) need to eat a variety of foods. Fruits and vegetables are especially important. Health experts recommend that we eat at least five servings of fruits and vegetables every day to live a healthier life and reduce the risk of cancer and other chronic diseases. Help get your children hooked on this habit early by offering a variety of choices throughout the day. The table below outlines what your child needs for a balanced diet that provides the right amount of calories and nutrients:

Groups of Foods	What They Need Per Day	One Serving Could Be**
Fruits	2 or more servings including at least 1 vitamin C source	1 medium piece of fruit, such as apple, orange, or banana; ¾ cup juice; ½ cup cooked fruit
Vegetables	3 or more servings	1 cup leafy salad greens; ½ cup cooked vegetable
Grains	6 or more servings	1 ounce ready-to-eat breakfast cereal; 1 slice whole-grain bread; ½ cup cooked rice, pasta, or cereal; 4 to 6 crackers; 1 tortilla, muffin, or dinner roll; ½ bagel or hamburger bun
Milk,* Cheese, Yogurt	4 servings	1 cup low-fat or nonfat milk or yogurt; 1½ ounces cheese
Meat, Fish, Poultry, Beans, Eggs, and Nuts	2 to 3 servings	2 to 4 ounces cooked, lean meat, fish, or chicken. Substitute 1 egg; ½ cup cooked peas or beans; or 2 tablespoons peanut butter for 1 ounce of meat.
Fats, Oils, and Sweets	Go easy on these foods and beverages.	

*Children under 2 years of age should drink whole milk.
**Younger children may eat smaller serving sizes.

Chart II
TOTAL CALORIES
RECOMMENDED PER DAY

Note: The "average calories needed" are based on RDA guidelines and fulfill recommended daily allowances.

Category	Age (years)	Average Weight (pounds)	Average Height (inches)	Average Calories Needed
Children	1 to 3	29	35	1,300
	4 to 6	44	44	1,800
	7 to 10	62	52	2,000
Males	11 to 14	99	62	2,500
	15 to 18	145	69	3,000
Females	11 to 14	101	62	2,200
	15 to 18	120	64	2,200

OUR FAVORITE FOOD CHOICES

For children over age two, our favorite food choices are low in saturated fat and cholesterol. Low-fat milk, low-fat ice cream and yogurt, low-fat cheeses, lean meats, poultry, and fish—these are all excellent sources of protein, iron, zinc, and calcium needed to support good growth.

A good example of "the varied diet" can be seen in the choices of a typical fourteen-year-old boy who eats a bagel with margarine and orange juice for breakfast; a turkey sandwich, some carrot sticks, chocolate milk, and a piece of chocolate cake for lunch; two microwave pizzas for a snack after school; french fries, a hamburger, two glasses of milk, cucumber slices, and cookies for dinner; and a Popsicle and orange soda before bed. Many of the foods on this menu are "high" in fat, many are low. When eaten together and varied from day to day, they effectively provide this youngster with good nutrition to meet his needs.

Snacks and snack foods (see page 116) are a necessary part of a child's diet and if they are varied to include fruits and vegetables and foods from the main food groups—and not just cookies, cakes, and candy bars—they can effectively complement meals in supplying good nutrition.

WHERE THEY GET THEIR VITAMINS

As stated, children who are on their growth curve and who eat a balanced diet do not routinely need vitamin supplements. This applies to children whose eating patterns are erratic (see page 148).

A ready supply of the foods from the various food groups, as suggested in the chart above, will supply children with the vitamins that they need.

Fruits and Vegetables These foods—including fresh, frozen, canned, or dried fruits, vegetables, and their juices—are rich in the B vitamins, folate, iron, and vitamins A and C.

Grains Including breads, muffins, cereals, rice, noodles, and pasta, grains are high in thiamine, niacin, vitamin B_6; magnesium, zinc (if whole grain), and iron (if fortified).

Dairy Products Dairy products—including whole and low-fat milk, buttermilk, yogurt, cheese, cottage cheese, ice cream, custard, and pudding—are high in protein, calcium, vitamins A and D, and riboflavin.

Meat, Poultry, Fish, and Beans These foods, including eggs, are good sources of protein, iron, zinc, copper, vitamins B_6 and B_{12}, and niacin.

(Grains, vegetables, and fresh fruits also supply fiber, which, while not a nutrient, contributes to normal bowel function.)

BOOSTING VITAMIN AWARENESS

Research increasingly shows the many subtle ways in which vitamins affect health, revealing quite a different view from what we have had of them in the past. For example, we know that vitamin A and vitamin E interfere with the oxidation of cholesterol in the blood vessels and thus can retard the development of certain toxic products of cholesterol that injure the blood vessel. They also appear to be somewhat beneficial in protecting against cancer in the colon, and perhaps in boosting immunity in some children to illnesses, such as measles.

This does not mean we should take vitamin E and A three times a day, but instead, it underscores the benefits of a diet that includes some fruits, vegetables, and other foods that contain these vitamins.

Iron is another example of the new findings. We used to think that if a youngster was not anemic, he or she did not need to pay that much attention to iron in the diet. Although it is controversial, there are case control studies that suggest that anemia is probably a late stage of iron deficiency and that early iron deficiency can result in learning difficulty and attention difficulty in children. Children who are iron deficient or who have diets that are deficient in iron but who are not grossly anemic (that is, who have hematocrits around 32 or 33 percent and who persist at that level) may have a higher prevalence of these problems. It is not known what contribution iron deficiency makes, however, to learning disabilities and attention deficit hyperactivity disorder.

Once again, this is not to overemphasize iron or make a case for iron tablets. Rather, it underscores the need for foods that supply iron in a child's diet, which could include "iron-fortified" foods and drinks, an easy way to help ensure iron quotas.

In this respect, iron fortification of infant formulas and cereals has brought iron levels up to normal in bottle-fed babies at a crucial time of growth. Fortification shows the public health approach to be effective—rather than give iron pills to every baby in the United States, introducing it in formula has proved to be a valuable boost to the population. Breakfast cereal and pasta are two of the items that are now iron fortified. Vitamin C has been added to apple juice; calcium has been added to orange juice, although in the latter case, no one knows yet what impact that will make on bones or the overall nutritional status of American children.

Iron in the Varied Diet To help ensure good iron stores and increase iron absorption in children, provide the following:

- Sufficient calories to maintain weight. A normal varied diet contains approximately 5 to 6 milligrams of iron for each 1,000 calories supplied. If insufficient calories are consumed, it is very likely that insufficient iron will be consumed.
- Vitamin C foods at meals (vitamin C increases iron absorption).
- Breads, pastas, and cereals that are "enriched" or "fortified with iron."
- Lean red meats, dark-meat chicken, dark-meat turkey. Animal protein contains iron as heme, the most readily absorbed form of iron (40 percent absorption in the gastrointestinal tract, versus 10 percent or less absorption for nonheme iron).

Vitamin D and Calcium An eight-ounce glass of milk supplies about 300 milligrams of calcium; 800 milligrams of calcium a day is the recommended daily allowance for a child under age eleven. Milk also supplies vitamin D, which helps the body absorb and retain calcium; vitamin A, important for maintaining eyesight and protecting mucous membranes; and phosphorus, which along with calcium, is important for strong bones.

After age two, skim or low-fat milk is recommended. If a

Some Children's Foods That Are High in Iron

Food	Serving Size	Iron Content (in milligrams)
Raisins	⅔ cup	2.1
Hamburger	3.5 ounces	3.0
Cream of Wheat	¾ cup, cooked	9.0
Oatmeal	¾ cup, cooked	8.1
Eggs	1, large	1.0
Chicken	3.5 ounces	1.1 to 1.5
Baked Beans	½ cup	2.1
Chili, Vegetarian	1 cup	4.0

NOTE: *Vitamin C (e.g., orange juice) increases iron absorption when taken with foods such as these listed.*

child likes to have three glasses of milk a day, that's fine, but other dairy products can serve as food equivalents—low-fat cheese, yogurt, and frozen desserts, for instance. Any solid form of milk (for example, cheese) in which water content is reduced provides a concentrated form of calcium. You can usually see this by checking labels and comparing the amount of calcium in an ounce of hard cheese as compared with the calcium in an ounce of soft cheese or other soft-consistency dairy product.

Many children do not like milk, but they do like pizza or macaroni and cheese, and these are usually loaded with cheese. Some children will not drink plain milk, but enjoy it flavored.

Lactase deficiency results in a low tolerance to milk. This occurs in almost everyone as they get older, and is often more of a problem in dark-skinned children at an early age. For example, about 50 percent of African-American four-year-olds have lactase deficiency, and when they get to about age ten, that percentage is probably closer to 90 to 100 percent. The milk that accompanies their school lunches, therefore, may cause cramps, bloating, or diarrhea (for them, juice or another nonmilk beverage or lactase-treated milk would be preferable).

Lactase deficiency does not immediately require a calcium supplement as there are several factors a pediatrician will consider first to decide whether a child is at risk. These include problems that might show up on the growth curve and whether or not the child was getting enough calcium and vitamin D from other parts of his or her diet besides milk.

If a child were falling off their growth curve, then the pediatrician would start thinking more aggressively about whether he or she was getting enough calcium and vitamin D, and whether the problem was really caused by a lactase deficiency.

The idea of packing the bones with calcium at a young age so there is less risk of osteoporosis in later years remains to be proven, and there are other factors besides an adequate supply of calcium that also have a role in how well bones are mineralized—namely, genetics, hormones (as exemplified by estrogen use in women), and physical exercise.

In any case, black people with lactase deficiency are at no greater risk for osteoporosis than anyone else because they are very efficient at mineralizing the bones—more efficient than people who are light skinned. This has been shown by a comparison of the bone density of adolescents, with the bone density for dark-skinned people being greater than that for light-skinned people. Osteoporosis is also much less common among older black women than older white-skinned women.

More Vitamin-Rich Food Sources As the following table shows, many foods that children enjoy are rich in the vitamins that children and adolescents need for growth.

The sample menus on pages 149–151—geared to show that erratic eating habits do not affect vitamin intake in a child's overall diet—also illustrate how a varied diet provides children with adequate amounts of vitamins and minerals.

Vitamin C	Vitamin A	Iron	Calcium	Zinc	Vitamin B$_{12}$
Apples	Milk, cheese,	Egg yolks	Cottage cheese,	Red meats	Dairy products
Cantaloupe	and other	Red meats	yogurt, and	Poultry	Eggs
Citrus Fruits:	dairy	Organ meats	other dairy	Organ meats	Seafood
Oranges	products	(e.g., liver)	products	Seafood	Meat
Grapefruits	Meats	Enriched,	Dark green,	Eggs	
Tangerines	Tuna fish	whole-grain	leafy	Whole grains	
Lemons	Cantaloupe	bread and	vegetables*	Milk	
Strawberries	Peaches	cereals*	Collard greens		
Cabbage	Yellow squash	Dried beans and	Broccoli		
Asparagus	Spinach	peas (lentils)	Kale		
Broccoli	Plums	Dried fruits:	Mustard		
Cauliflower	Asparagus	Apricots	greens		
Spinach	Broccoli	Raisins	Spinach		
Kale	Carrots	Dates	Tuna fish		
Kiwi	Spinach	Prunes	Salmon with		
Turnips	Kale	Figs	bones		
Leafy, green	Turnips	Greens and	Sardines		
vegetables	Tomatoes	leafy	Dried beans		
Potatoes	Winter squash	vegetables	and peas		
Tomatoes	Green peppers	Kale	Citrus fruits		
Green peppers	Pumpkin	Chard			
Red peppers	Sweet potatoes	Spinach			
		Potatoes			

*The ability to absorb or actually use (bioavailability) iron from grains and vegetables and calcium from vegetables may vary significantly.

SNACKS AS A SOURCE OF NUTRITION

We concur with the opinion of most nutritionists and pediatricians that having snacks is a good way for children to keep up with the calories and nutrients they need for growth. Children get hungrier faster than adults—their stomachs are small for the energy they expend, and they need food every few hours.

Left to their own inclinations to eat when they are hungry, children will get 35 percent of their calories and nutrients from the snacks they eat during the day.

Breakfast, snack; lunch, snack; dinner, snack—this is the typical eating pattern that continues throughout childhood, especially during phases when growth is active.

Observe the typical, on-the-go adolescent boy and girl—

they graze all day long and do not seem to gain weight. If you restrict their eating, teenagers (or children of any age, for that matter) get very mean, tell you all day long that they are hungry, or lose weight—something that should definitely *not* occur with normal children, especially in adolescence, when growth activity is intense.

Accepting the idea of snacking makes it much easier to live with a child who does not consume an ideal breakfast, lunch, or dinner. The knowledge that snacking gives children multiple opportunities to meet their daily nutrition needs can really help to take the pressure off of what goes down at mealtimes. If food intake at some meals is picky, snacks over the course of the day can make up for the missed calories.

Should snacks be limited? It depends. In keeping with the idea that a child's appetite is cued by hunger and that he or she should have ready access to food, we do not recommend withholding or limiting food when children say they are hungry. The child's age is a consideration, however, as well as how close the demand for food is to mealtime. Obviously, a crying, hungry three-month-old or six-month-old child needs to be fed right away, but an eight-year-old who wants food at five-thirty when dinner will be on the table at six can be held off until then, or given some raw vegetables in the interim.

The key is not to fight about withholding food, especially when a child is tired and cranky and demands it. In that case, especially if the child has not eaten for a few hours, having something to eat will boost his or her sense of well-being and security, and make that child easier to live with.

On the other hand, if a highly processed snack food is eaten to the exclusion of everything else—for example, if potato chips (which are high in fat) are the only vegetable a child eats every day—that's not a very balanced diet. Children need to know that. They need to know that there is nothing wrong with potato chips or soda or candy bars or any other high-fat food as snacks as long as other, more nutritious foods are also treated as snacks. Steady snacking on low-nutrition foods may satisfy hunger but it does not provide children with the nutrients they need for activities and growth.

Presented with this information, most children will choose to balance out high- and low-nutrition snack foods and set their own snacking limits. (See also Chapter 12, "Resolving the Junk Food Dilemma.")

What to Supply for Between-Meal Nutrition If you think of snacks as providing between-meal nutrition, then any kind of food that supplies a mixture of nutrients is a good snack. Apple juice, orange juice, milk, chocolate milk, saltines, graham crackers, bananas, apple slices, carrot sticks, fresh raw string beans, cookies or cupcakes—if it's Johnny's birthday snack at school—these are all fine snacks as long as they are age appropriate, i.e., can be managed without choking.

Potato chips, soda, or processed snack foods can also be included, if, as mentioned, other high-nutrition snacks are served to balance out the child's diet.

Beverages Make Great Snacks Beverages are an excellent source of nutrition, at the same time supplying the fluids children need to maintain a healthy body. Children enjoy drinks as snacks because they go down quickly, can be handled sitting or standing, and do not stop them from pursuing activities. Most children will drink whenever they are thirsty—on average, taking in about one to two quarts of fluid a day in four-ounce to eight-ounce servings. Thus it makes good sense to have a variety of beverages on hand, and to suggest them as snacks.

Milk Three eight-ounces glasses (or the equivalent in smaller servings) supply children up to age eleven with the recommended daily allowance of calcium. Most children enjoy milk or flavored milk as a snack—chocolate, coffee, or strawberry—mixing it up themselves.

Fruit Juices One eight-ounce glass of orange or grapefruit juice supplies a child with some potassium as well as his or her daily requirement of vitamin C (60 milligrams a day over six months of age). Tomato juice supplies vitamin C, potassium, and also vitamin A (30 to 70 percent of the RDA). Two eight-ounce servings of juice a day is more than adequate.

Fruit-flavored drinks; caffeine-free herbal tea; or an occasional soda do not supply important nutrients, but they do supply fluids and they are certainly acceptable as part of a varied diet.

Combination Drinks For highly nutritious snacks, combine fresh fruits or vegetables in a blender or juicer—for example, a combination of banana slices, strawberries, yogurt, and orange or pineapple juice whipped up in a blender, with a tablespoon of wheat germ stirred in and a spritz of seltzer. Children enjoy helping with preparation.

SNACK TIPS AND SUGGESTIONS

- Look at snacking as another way besides meals for your child to get nutrients during the day.
- Recognize the importance of snacking in supplying energy throughout the day; a child's body is not equipped to store large amounts of energy beyond a couple of hours.
- Make sure your child has ready access to a wide variety of snack foods: fresh fruits and vegetables, vitamin-enriched drinks, cheese, chips, popcorn, cookies, etc.
- Make meal foods, for example, small boxes of packaged breakfast cereal, as much a part of snacking as candy or soda.
- Offer children fluids after activities, especially when the weather is hot. Offer them plain cold water first, followed by a choice of beverages.
- For avoiding conflicts over snacks, see page 169.

SPECIAL CONSIDERATIONS

The Five-a-Day Guideline According to the National Cancer Institute (NCI) and the U.S. Department of Health and Human Services, populations consuming diets rich in fruits and vegetables, particularly those rich in vitamins A (beta carotene) and C, have significantly lower rates of cancer of the colon, breast, lung, oral cavity, larynx, esophagus, stomach, bladder, and pancreas.

The National Cancer Institute and other health agencies encourage the consumption of five servings of a variety of fruits and vegetables every day for better health. These health organizations agree that the benefits of consuming fruits and vegetables every day far outweigh any potential risk from possible exposure to pesticide residues (see Chapter 1, "Is It Safe?" and also page 269 for ordering brochures on food safety from the NCND).

As illustrated in Chart I, page 109, by the number of recommended servings, we endorse the idea of providing the five-a-day quota of fruits and vegetables in a child's diet, as well as in an adult's diet—applied not as a strict rule but rather as a loose guideline to help keep the daily intake of less nutritious foods in balance. On average, five a day is not really all that much to provide over the course of a day. Adding them up, it could be a banana (1) with cereal; lettuce (2) and tomato (3) on a sandwich; potatoes (4) as part of dinner; and (5) an apple or plum or some other piece of fruit as a snack.

When they are included as snacks, fruits and vegetables can help satisfy a child's need for nutritious, between-meal foods without excluding candy bars or other snack choices.

The Food Guide Pyramid and Children Inasmuch as it emphasizes the "varied food message," the USDA "food guide pyramid" is clearly beneficial. Clearly, it helps adults implement the idea of making healthy food choices and yet, in our opinion, the food pyramid has not made a major impact on childhood nutrition. In fact, there is some concern among nutrition experts that the negative emphasis on the use of meat and dairy products will be taken to an extreme or misinterpreted by parents to think these foods should be avoided.

When parents ask us about it, we suggest to them that the best way to use the pyramid is to do their best in increasing the consumption of fresh fruit and vegetables in the family, but not necessarily to decrease the consumption of meat, poultry, and dairy products.

Vegetarian Diets and Children Children whose parents' or whose personal tastes and preferences tend toward a nonmeat or vegetarian diet can obtain adequate protein and vitamins for growth from a variety of "food combinations"—that is, foods that, when eaten together in a meal, serve as a complete protein source. There are any number of appetizing, nutritious dishes that can boost these food combinations.

For example:

- *Legumes with grains (including peanuts and beans)*. Rice with beans, peanut butter in a sandwich or on crackers, enchiladas with beans and sauce.
- *Grains or other vegetable protein with milk*. Cold and hot cereals with milk, rice pudding, vegetable lasagna, macaroni and cheese, breakfast breads made with milk.
- *Legumes with seeds or nuts*. For example, hummus (chickpea and sesame seed paste).
- *Grains or other vegetable protein with eggs*. Quiche, fried rice, pound cake, pancakes, waffles, rice pudding.

10

• • • •

A Child-Oriented
Approach to
Fitness and Exercise

Many parents worry about whether their child is in good shape physically—whether he or she is "sitting around too much," not getting enough exercise, or "falling behind" with sports skills. Media reports on declining fitness levels in children do not help to alleviate these concerns; if anything, they put more pressure on parents to get their children involved in organized sports and competitive activities at increasingly younger ages, often before they are physically ready. For the child, this can be dangerous as well as discouraging.

According to recommendations made by the American Academy of Pediatrics, children need a minimum of half an hour of sustained aerobic exercise three times a week in order to meet fitness requirements—a standard that the majority of children can easily meet.

Children seldom commit to exercise and fitness as intensely as adults do. They pursue physical activities to have fun—that's their prime motivation. If parents do nothing else for their child in this area, *they should strive to keep the fun in fitness activities,* helping their child find the balance between sports, fitness, and fun from which they will benefit.

A three-step approach, as detailed in this chapter, can help accomplish this goal:

1. Become an informed parent—learn about fitness and its benefits; evaluate your child's individual situation and special needs.

2. Share in your child's activities—find ways to maximize fun together.

3. Reinforce fitness with a varied diet.

What Is Physical Fitness?

Physical fitness relates to the level of energy that allows the human body to carry out daily tasks, pursue leisure activities, maintain peak intellectual efficiency, and enjoy life. Physical fitness is most often measured by two components: health-related fitness and skill-related fitness.

Health-Related Fitness Five factors contribute to health-related fitness: (1) *cardiorespiratory, or aerobic, endurance,* the ability of the heart and lungs to circulate oxygen and nutrients to body tissues and to perform and recover from tasks—the element considered to be the most important component of fitness; (2) *body composition,* or the percentage of fat that makes up total body weight; (3) *muscle strength,* or the maximum amount of force that can be exerted by a muscle or muscles against a resistance in a single effort; (4) *muscle endurance,* or ability of the muscles to exert force repeatedly or sustain a contraction for a given length of time; and (5) *flexibility,* or the ability of muscles and joints to move through their full range of motion.

Skill-Related Fitness This includes *agility,* the ability to change direction with speed and accuracy; *balance,* the ability to maintain equilibrium while the body is stationary or moving; *coordination,* the use of the senses to perform motor tasks easily and accurately; *speed,* the ability to perform a movement or task within a short period of time; *power,* the ability to perform work at a specific rate; and *reaction time,* the ability to respond quickly to a stimulus.

The Three Benefits of Exercise for Children

Fitness and activity make valuable contributions in three areas in childhood: *growth and physical development,* as outlined above; *socialization,* by promoting teamwork and cooperation; and the *increase in self-esteem.* The ability to master skills, to run, to be part of a team, to show strength and coordination, gives children the confidence to try new challenges and risk failure. In addition, as good nutrition helps performance and increases physical capabilities, children who feel good about their body being in good shape are more inclined to make healthy food choices starting at a young age.

For all these benefits, children should be encouraged to participate in activities that provide sustained, aerobic exercise. This is possible by selecting a variety of activities for exercise and active play. Keep in mind that (1) some physical activity every day is desirable; (2) it can be in the house or out of the house; and (3) it should be fun.

Organized sports such as baseball and soccer offer one opportunity for the child to participate in aerobic exercise and stay fit, but so do everyday activities such as running and climbing in the playground, biking, jumping rope, roller skating, or playing tag. On weekends, activities such as skating, Frisbee, a family soccer game, or simply taking a walk together can be both purposeful and fun.

Evaluating Your Child's Situation

Evaluate your child's routines and activities, particularly at school or away from your care, to determine whether the recommended requirements are currently being met. Look at his or her activity levels within the context of a well-rounded childhood. Is what you see as "a sedentary life-style" merely a well-deserved break in a highly active day, during which your child easily fulfills the recommendations for aerobic exercise?

Arrange a meeting with the physical educator at your child's school to gain an understanding of the program's goals and characteristics. An effective physical education program offers activities to develop physical fitness, and it provides opportunities for skill development in games, gymnastics, rhythm, and dance activities.

Coaches and Physical Educators The role of the coach or physical educator is all-important; parents should take steps to ensure that the coach/instructor relationship will be a positive experience for a child. Choose after-school and team activities carefully, taking into consideration the qualifications of the coach or group leader. Before committing to an after-school or weekend sports team, watch from the sidelines for a few games to see how the coach interacts with the team players—whether the coach knows how to coach, can keep his or her ego in check, and encourages the players to have fun with their peers while improving skills. Childhood injuries can occur when the coach is untrained in proper skill techniques and methods of training.

Talk with the coach and other parents whose children play on the team. Are the goals of the team appropriate for the youngsters' age, without pushing them beyond their capabilities or putting them under pressure?

Fitness Choices:
Matching Activities to Ability

For their enjoyment and safety, children should be free to choose a variety of sports and activities that are geared to their age, ability, and interest. That way they can discover what they like best. Some children are drawn to team sports and enjoy socializing within the group; others are drawn to sports that develop individual skills.

Whatever they choose, encourage them to progress at their own rate. Remind them (and yourself) that in pursuing various activities, the goal is to have fun, not to strive for perfection or to start an argument. Parents who drive a child too hard run the risk of taking the fun out of the game or the activity. Children often burn out as a result of too much too soon. Pushed into sports too early or discouraged about their skills, they will drop out of activity or exercise they might otherwise have enjoyed.

If your child decides not to continue in a sport, discuss the situation and see if you can help, but let him or her know you support the decision. If not pressured into staying with it, children frequently will return to a sport or activity later on, even after leaving it for a while. Sometimes problems that involve skills can be solved before children drop out (see "Breaking the Cycle of Self-Defeat," page 133).

Competition While it appears that some children are able to understand elements related to competition as early as age three or four, the ability to understand what it means to perform better than another child does not indicate their readiness for competitive activities in an adult fashion. Most pediatricians and sports-related experts share the opinion that children younger than age five or six do not have the ability to learn the skills needed to perform in organized sports.

Between ages five and ten years, children should be exposed to a variety of cooperative sports and activities—not to prepare them for competition or compare their abilities, but to give them positive associations.

Between ages eleven and fifteen, children become physically and mentally ready for the increased training and practice time needed to develop proper techniques. As children enter puberty at different ages, there will be major differences between them in size and abilities.

Are They Physically Ready to Play?

Unfortunately, some parents will coax their children to perform activities beyond their physical ability, without realizing that they need to develop skill-related fitness before participating in organized games. The prerequisites for any sport or activity include the identification of body parts, managing the body through obstacles, moving at different speeds, and manipulating objects. Other skills to be mastered include *locomotor movements*—walking, running, hopping, jumping, skipping, galloping, sliding, and leaping; and *nonlocomotor movements*—bending, straightening, stretching, falling, swaying, swinging, twisting, and turning.

Children develop competence at physical skills gradually. In rough chronological order, here are some average age ranges:

- *Reaching, grasping, and releasing at will* (from primitive reaching behaviors to controlled grasp-and-release skills): from two months to eighteen months.
- *Throwing* (from ball thrown with forearm extension only to mature throwing pattern): from two years to six years and over.
- *Catching* (from chasing a large ball on the ground, to catching a small ball in the air, using hands only): from two years to five years.
- *Kicking* (from pushing against the ball with legs and feet, to mature pattern of kicking through the ball): from eighteen months to six years.

- *Striking* (i.e., contact with objects in an overarm, sidearm, or underhand pattern, from facing the object and swinging on a vertical plane, to rotating the trunk and hips and shifting the body weight forward to achieve mature horizontal striking patterns): from two years to seven years.
- *Dynamic Balance* (i.e., maintaining equilibrium as the center of gravity shifts, from walking a one-inch straight line, to walking on a three-inch beam, to performing a mature forward roll): from three years to seven years.
- *Static Balance* (i.e., maintaining equilibrium while the center of gravity remains stationary): from pulling to a standing position (ten months), to standing alone (twelve months), to balancing on one foot for three to five seconds (five years), to supporting the body in basic inverted positions (six years).
- *Axial movements* (i.e., static postures that involve bending, stretching, twisting, turning, etc.): from two months to six years, gradually being incorporated into coordinated patterns of throwing, catching, striking, trapping, and other activities.

Readiness Guidelines for Sports and Activities

For a child's enjoyment and safety, popular activities and sports should be properly matched to his or her competence in skills and stage of development.

BASEBALL/SOFTBALL

Introducing children to the game with oversized plastic bats and balls will give them a sense of accomplishment and at the same time ensure safety.

T-ball, which can be played with children as young as three years old, is an excellent method for introducing young children to batting skills. The ball is placed on an adjustable batting tee, and the child can practice batting techniques with a very high rate of success. As the child gains skill (from age six and older), underhand and then overhand pitching can be used.

Nine- and ten-year-olds are usually ready for real baseballs or softballs; however, at first, baseball skills should be practiced with soft baseballs, soft softballs, and light bats.

Throwing and catching skills can be introduced as early as age two; however, these skills do not mature until about age six. To avoid injuries to a child's arm, pitching requires expert coaching. Children should not pitch regularly until they are at least nine years old. To keep the game moving as children develop skills, parents should pitch and catch.

BASKETBALL

Children can begin to participate in basketball at age six, with simple skill challenges. Miniature foam basketballs and adjustable rims help give the young child a feeling of success in making a basket.

BIKING

With consistent practice time, children ages three and above can develop proficiency on a tricycle or four-wheel bike. With consistent practice time, children ages five and above can develop proficiency on a two-wheel bike. (Once again *practice time* is the key.)

All children who ride a bike should wear bike helmets; so should their parents.

Correct proportion of child to bike is essential for balance and control—the bike should be small enough and the seat in the proper position so that the child's feet can easily reach the ground.

GYMNASTICS

Children can begin participating in gymnastics programs at age six; preparation for gymnastics can actually be earlier than that, in toddler or preschool programs. These programs should be properly supervised and emphasize fun.

When choosing a gymnastics program, parents should inquire about the nutritional philosophy of the teacher. If he or she overemphasizes thinness as an integral part of the program, this can negatively influence a child's eating patterns.

ICE SKATING

The balance required for ice skating does not develop until around age five or six, although some children younger than that will want to try to skate. That's fine; enjoyment is the key. However, if a child falls repeatedly during the initial skating experience, he or she will inevitably become discouraged. For this reason, lessons from a qualified instructor and a good pair of skates are a wise investment. Poorly fitting skates can cause sore ankles and added frustration.

JUDO AND KARATE

Children as young as age six can participate in judo and karate, provided the coach is very well qualified and experienced in working with children. Overtraining or improper training can result in serious injury.

POOL SWIMMING

Pool activity and swimming lessons require very close adult supervision. Children can be introduced to shallow-water activities (no deeper than one foot) as early as six months. These activities can include games that involve walking in the water, sitting in the water and kicking feet, splashing, and tapping the surface of the water—but always with an adult holding on to them.

Most children are ready for swimming lessons (from a qualified instructor) between the ages of three and five, but children should not be pushed into learning how to swim until they overcome any fears they may have of the water. Parents who are competent swimmers can act as role models in the water—helping build their child's confidence by showing him or her that swimming is fun.

Some children have the physical ability to begin competitive swimming in grade school, but developmentally, a more realistic age to start competing would be around age twelve. With competitive swimming, it is important that the emphasis be on fun and fitness, not on winning at all cost.

SOCCER

Although attempts at primitive kicking (more like pushing) usually begin around eighteen months, the kicking skills needed for soccer are not fully developed until around age five or six, when children can be introduced to a noncompetitive version of the game with a soft soccer ball and emphasis on teamwork and skills. Field orientation in soccer changes as children mature. This is true in all sports. Five-year-olds playing soccer move in a clump all over the field, following the ball together. Seven- or eight-year-olds comprehend the difference between offense and defense moves; and at twelve or thirteen, they have a fully developed sense of working together as a team, adjusting their positions to other positions.

TENNIS

Children are capable of striking skills as early as age two; however, these skills do not mature until age five or six and even then the child may not have the ability to move to the ball to hit it properly. To increase control, children should use a lightweight racket with a large racket face.

VOLLEYBALL

Very young children can be introduced to "Newcomb," a lead-up game to volleyball that involves throwing and catching a beach ball over a net. Most nine- and ten-year-olds have the necessary skills to begin practicing real volleyball—at first, also using a beach ball. This allows them enough time to follow the ball visually, to move toward the ball, and to play the ball successfully. Oversized soft "training volleyballs" may be used as the child improves skills.

WEIGHT TRAINING

Children under the age of sixteen should not "weight train" as there is too great a risk of permanent damage to the growth plates of the bones (epiphysis). Prior to age sixteen, children can participate in a program of calisthenics, stretching, and strengthening. After age sixteen, it is important that the adolescent who wants to use weights work with a qualified trainer who will not be too aggressive with his or her training, and who will guide the adolescent in following a balanced diet. (For dietary cautions involving muscle building, see also page 138.)

A Child's Special Needs

Sports Tutoring Children who come to certain sports later than their peers, or who have limited skills and less practice time, tend to have limited participation in the activity. Parents of these children should work with the physical education teacher or the team coach to identify which skills the child should spend additional time practicing. It is important to take action that will guarantee at least some change in the child's abilities, as improvement brings with it a new level of confidence and a desire to participate more.

"Sports tutoring" is an effective way to strengthen skills, particularly if a parent is unable to get involved for practice time. Enlisting a high school player to work with the child over the summer or just prior to the sports season, or contacting a local college that trains physical educators or certifies coaches and arranging for the child to work with a recommended individual on a one-to-one basis can really work to a child's advantage.

Breaking the Cycle of Self-Defeat A pattern of self-defeat can emerge when a child refuses to participate in physical activities or sports because the child feels inept or awkward about his or her skills, weight, or appearance. This can be a big problem by the time a child is ten or eleven years old, particularly if he or she is slightly overweight (not unusual in prepubertal children today) because by then the child will have lost ground in his or her level of strength, stamina, and competence among peers, and a vicious cycle can begin. The last thing that child needs is pressure from parents, and yet that is what typically emerges. In the desire to see their child thinner, or more proficient in skills, parents may push for sports and exercise, and focus attention on the child's food. There are several things a parent can do to help in such a situation:

- Encourage the child not to be too hard on him- or herself—not to expect too much too soon from an activity the child wants to excel in. Encourage him or her to pursue the activity for fun now, not for future triumphs such as winning the U.S. Open.
- Do not be condescending or critical. Speak to your child in the same tone of voice you use with friends.

- Do not suddenly pressure the child to perform at sports or organized activities.
- Establish fitness goals together. Be willing to change your life-style, if need be, to meet them.
- Do not all at once drastically increase activity levels. Make small changes at first. Increase your child's opportunities for daily activities. Walk rather than drive, when that's possible, and encourage the use of stairs rather than elevators.
- Offer sports tutoring.
- Emphasize nutritious foods that are low in fat and sugar. Encourage your child to eat three nutritious meals a day, and to cut back on television time or video games to allow more time for exercise and physical activity.

Pursuing Fitness with Your Child

Getting involved early on in physical activities with your child is one of the best ways to show him or her that exercise can be fun. Whatever sport or activity you choose to do together, the experience has got to be mutually enjoyable, the atmosphere relaxed.

Select short-term goals and modified activities when sharing fitness activities. Soft foam balls, adjustable basketball rims, batting trees, and other equipment will increase the opportunities for the child to have fun and meet realistic goals; goals and equipment can be changed as the child becomes more skilled and his or her level of fitness increases.

Outdoor Activities Sedentary parents who expect their preadolescent child to be sports oriented should try to begin a program of jogging with them. Start with a simple five-minute run for several blocks, and gradually increase running time. Do not be surprised if your child's pace is beyond your own (yes, this can happen with walking, jogging, or bicycling, especially when that child is an adolescent). Don't push yourself. Look at it this way: You're giving your child's self-esteem a big boost by "letting" him or her outrun you.

If you are very athletic, adjust to your child's pace and assume that he or she will progress naturally, without excessive coaching. Some eight-year-old children, for example, can successfully run a mile at a good pace, while others must stop and walk intermittently. If you are running ten kilometers a day to train for a marathon, be aware that this is not an appropriate or safe distance for a child under the age of sixteen. Scale down the intensity and duration of your workout so that your child can participate with you. Your own exercise patterns may be excessive or even detrimental for the child's body. Except under very unusual circumstances, a child does not have the endurance, strength, or calories in his or her diet to perform at adult levels of training. Most adult activities put enormous stress on developing muscles and can even cause joint deterioration or permanent damage to the bones by inhibiting their growth.

These cautions are especially true for parents who participate in weight training activities, which are not recommended for children under age fifteen. With weights, the emphasis should always be on technique, rather than increasing the amount of weight.

Nutrition for Young Athletes

Reinforce your child's fitness goals by providing him or her with a full, varied diet. The informed parent who shares in the child's fitness activities and eats a balanced diet is in the ideal position to emphasize the correlation between eating nutritious, low-fat foods and getting a good workout or sports performance.

Keeping Up with Calorie Requirements

Athletic children need to eat what all children eat—only more. Physical exercise and activity justify more calories in the diet—larger quantities of food, more snacks, and as fat is the body's most abundant energy source, less concern about limiting fat. The amount of calories expended on exercise is about 1 to 3 calories per pound for every half hour of exercise, depending on the type of activity involved (see chart on next page).

The child's natural appetite cues him or her to eat more to make up for calories lost in activity. Observe your own child to see how increased physical activity increases hunger. At the end of an afternoon running around in the park, swimming in the lake or pool with friends, ice skating, or playing soccer your child will be ravenous and consume more food. As a snack, for example, the child who is not much of an athlete might have one Twinkie (yes, we did say Twinkie) and fruit juice, whereas the active athlete might have two Twinkies, an apple, and some chocolate milk.

When combined with the calories consumed by growth, the food intake required by a very active child or adolescent involved in sports can easily surpass the needs of many adults. To repeat the example given earlier, a healthy adolescent boy who plays soccer or ice hockey in school may burn upwards of 4,000 calories a day as opposed to his office-working parent, who may burn less than 2,000 calories. Strenuous exercise during adolescence can increase caloric requirements by 25 percent. To make up for the large quantities of calories burned, up to 1,000 calories at a sitting may be needed—supplied in meals and in readily available, high-energy snack foods interspersed throughout the day. The sample menu on pages 139 and 140 shows how food intake must be increased to meet calorie requirements for a teenage athlete (see also "How to Increase Protein, Calories, and Nutrients," page 222):

Calories burned by a 77- or 132-pound person during 10 minutes of continuous activity.

Activity	Calories Burned in 10 Minutes	
	BODY WEIGHT	
	77 pounds (35 kg)	132 pounds (60 kg)
Basketball (game)	60	102
Cross-country skiing	23	72
Cycling (9.3 mph or 15 km/h)	36	60
Judo	69	118
Running (5 mph or 8 km/h)	60	90
Sitting (complete rest)	9	12
Soccer (game)	63	108
Swimming (30 m/min or 33 yd)		
breaststroke	34	58
freestyle	43	74
Tennis	39	66
Volleyball (game)	35	60
Walking		
2.5 mph or 4 km/h	23	34
3.7 mph or 6 km/h	30	43

kg = kilogram
mph = miles per hour
km = kilometer
m = meter

Modified from O. Bar-Or, *Pediatric Sports Medicine for the Practitioner* (New York: Springer-Verlag, 1983), pp. 349–50.
J. M. Ferguson, *Habits, Not Diets* (Palo Alto, CA: Bull Publishing Co., 1988). Used with permission.

Example:
13-Year-Old Male Athlete

Percentile	Caloric Requirement
95	4,648
50	3,218
5	2,431

Example:
13-Year-Old Female Athlete

Percentile	Caloric Requirement
95	4,094
50	2,811
5	2,077

Special Considerations

Fluid Replacement and Mineral Losses in Athletes The loss of minerals, particularly sodium and potassium, which are also known as electrolytes, is not a problem with young athletes. Heavy losses of minerals only occur when sweating is profuse and, in that case, sodium and potassium are easily replaced by eating a balanced diet and drinking appropriate fluids.

Fluid replacement in athletes should be aimed at replenishing water. Salt tablets should be avoided; they can be dangerous. Alternatively, some of the commercially available solutions (such as Gatorade) that are intended for drinking during hot weather and strenuous activity contain electrolytes and sugar and are appropriate as "sweat replacement" solutions.

Protein and Muscle Mass There is no documented proof that extra protein, by way of protein supplements, will increase muscle mass, strength, or physical performance. The average American diet with 15 percent of its calories consumed as

SAMPLE MENU
FOR THE TEENAGE ATHLETE

		Calories	Protein
BREAKFAST:			
1 cup grapefruit juice		80	
2 slices French toast		230	10
2 teaspoons margarine		90	
1 cup sweetened cereal		160	3
½ cup blueberries		40	
2 tablespoons sugar		80	
1 cup whole milk		160	8
	Total	840	21
LUNCH:			
1 cup whole milk		160	8
3 ounces hamburger		225	21
1 roll		140	3
2 slices American cheese		215	12
2 teaspoons mayonnaise		90	
lettuce, tomato, fried onions		25	
1 cup french fries		310	2
¼ cup catsup		60	
1 baked apple with ice cream		190	1
8 ounces cola		95	
	Total	1,510	47
DINNER:			
1 cup cream of chicken soup		180	1
5 ounces salmon,		275	35
cooked in butter		90	
½ cup creamed corn		160	1
½ cup zucchini in		25	1
tomato sauce		55	
2 dinner rolls		140	6
2 teaspoons margarine		90	
1 slice angel food cake		135	1
1 cup whole milk		160	8
	Total	1,310	53
AFTERNOON SNACK:			
1 slice pizza		145	18
with extra cheese		100	
1 cup chocolate milk		210	8
	Total	455	26

SAMPLE MENU
FOR THE TEENAGE ATHLETE—Continued

EVENING SNACK:

2 ounces chocolate-covered peanuts	320	2
8 ounces cola	95	
Total	415	2

WEIGHT: *143 pounds*
TOTAL CALORIES: *4,530/day*
TOTAL PROTEIN: *149 gm = 2.3 g. protein/kg/2.2 pounds, OR 1 g protein/pound*

protein is more than sufficient for maintaining vital body tissues. Adolescents and young athletes interested in body-building should know that improved muscle conditioning and performance is only achieved through repetitive exercise and genetic potential. Protein supplements can be harmful and expensive; they should be avoided.

Extra Vitamins For young athletes, children, and adolescents, extra vitamins are not necessary. Unless there is a known vitamin deficiency, as determined by a medical checkup, the balanced diet as outlined on page 109 together with good eating habits will provide all the nutrients needed for optimum athletic performance and growth.

Adolescents, particularly those who pursue sports, need to pay special attention to their eating habits. A steady diet of only a few foods, and poor eating habits (skipping meals), can lead to vitamin deficiencies—specifically, in this age group, of the B vitamins, calcium, iron, or zinc.

Putting Your Child's Needs First: A Fitness Checklist

- Work with other parents to ensure that there are regular physical education classes at your child's school, five times a week.

- Choose an after-school program on the basis of activities offered and the level of fun for children, not on whether they always have healthy snacks. If your child is old enough, let him or her share in choosing the after-school program.
- To help bring a child's skill levels up, encourage him or her to try out for a weekend sports team. If you are divorced, be sure that visitation schedules take a child's sports commitments and physical activities into account.
- Think about your own priorities. Be willing to compromise your time for your child's; for example, adjust weekend time so your child can participate in extracurricular seasonal activities such as soccer or Little League, if that is what he or she wants.
- Periodically review your child's changing needs. Is the child's physical activity and enjoyment of exercise on par with his or her age group? How does the child's activity fit within the context of family life and friendships, sense of self-esteem, and need for fun? You know your child best. Try to promote activities you know he or she will enjoy.
- Encourage the child to get involved in physical activities, but let the child choose what he or she wants to do.
- The "fit" between child and sport is important; help your child make a choice that will give him or her optimum satisfaction, depending on body type, interests, and attention span. For example, a child who has a short attention span may not last as long as a track meet lasts, whereas that same child may make an excellent goalie—he or she only needs a short time to concentrate on the ball, do what has to be done, and then relax for a while.

  Children who are physically more aggressive interpersonally often do very well in swimming, which can give them a sense of containment and competition.
- If your child does not like an activity after giving it a try,

let the child drop out but encourage him or her to join another.

- Don't make the child feel guilty for the time and money you may have spent on organized activities he or she no longer wants to do.
- If the child is into something that's over his or her head, let the child know it's okay with you if he or she wants to drop out for now and come back to the activity at a later stage.
- Meet with the child's coach or physical education instructor in school; become informed about his or her teaching methods and goals for your child.
- Help your child push through frustration and disappointment in learning new skills. Do not dismiss the child's sense of awkwardness or frustration—let him or her know that everyone feels awkward as a beginner. Give the child some examples of what he or she does well. Praise the child's progress and persistence.
- Look for ways to show the child that you aren't perfect either—ideally, that he or she can do better than you can in some things.
- Don't overdo practice time. Twenty minutes is ample time for any activity; more than that may take away from the fun.
- Be patient. It's natural for a child to test your reactions. If the child sees you get angry or impatient with his or her performance, it provides him or her with good enough reason to give up.
- Do not compare your child to other children (especially not to brothers and sisters), brag about your own past performances, or express disappointment in his or her choice of physical activity.
- Look to your own activities in setting an example for your child. If you are sedentary, do not expect your child to

pursue fitness with great zeal or enjoyment. Find a sport or activity you can enjoy together.

- Give the child ready access to nutritious snack foods and provide healthy food choices at mealtimes—in ample amounts when activity levels are high.

◆ ◆ ◆

Feeding Interactions and Conflicts over Food

11

❖   ❖   ❖   ❖

How to Keep
Mealtimes from
Driving You Crazy

The two-year-old child dawdles so long over breakfast that her bowl of cereal gets soggy; a second grader demands food an hour before and after picking at his dinner; a teenager finishes off in one afternoon all the snack foods purchased for the week . . . and parents throw up their hands in frustration.

When children follow their natural hunger cues, it can be a source of tension that every parent will recognize—and at the same time elicit reactions that may run counter to the children's needs.

Adults approach food and eating with conditioned responses that have been shaped by a complex variety of social, cultural, and psychological factors; what, how, and when they choose to eat are all largely determined by external cues. In comparison, a child's natural appetite is cued by hunger—the body's internal mechanism that tells the child to eat when his or her stomach is empty and to stop eating when it is full.

Both children and adults have hungry days and not-so-hungry days, but whether they are hungry or not, most adults will eat at regular, three-meal intervals spaced throughout the day. In contrast, children don't care whether eating times are defined as a meal or a snack or something else—responding to their hunger cue, they either need food immediately or do not need it at all. Picky eating, lack of appetite, boredom with food, ravenous hunger at odd times—these are all signs that a child is following internal cues that tell him or her when and how much to eat.

When a grown-up responds to what he or she sees as erratic eating by withholding food because "it's not time to eat" or coercing a child to eat a meal, that grown-up unwittingly sends a confusing message to the child. This in turn can lead to conflict, and that conflict can lead to any number of things—disobedience, passive behavior, sneaking food, and if it keeps building, to a whole variety of other problems, some of which may be food-related, some not. Much depends on how rigid the parent's attitude is about control issues such as food, and how rigid the child's attitude is in response.

Erratic Eating Is Normal

Despite life-style changes related to when families typically eat and what they eat, studies over the years have shown that the variable eating patterns of American children do not ultimately affect their nutritional status or the total calorie intake required for healthy growth.

A widely cited study was done by Leann Birch and her research colleagues at The Child Development Laboratory in Urbana, Illinois, the results of which were published in the *New England Journal of Medicine* in January 1991. Records were kept of the food eaten over the course of a week by fifteen children ranging in age from two to five. Amounts of food eaten varied widely from meal to meal. Sometimes the children hardly touched the food on their plates and sometimes they had seconds. In any case, they stopped eating when they were full. While the amount of calories these children ate varied from a few hundred calories in a meal to a thousand calories,

AGES 0–2

Day 1: Low Calorie	*Day 2: High Calorie*	*Day 3: Average*
BREAKFAST 6 ounces whole milk ½ blueberry muffin	6 A.M. 8 ounces whole milk	BREAKFAST ¾ cup oatmeal with cinnamon sugar 6 ounces whole milk
SNACK 2 ounces apple juice	BREAKFAST 2 pancakes with syrup and margarine 4 ounces whole milk	SNACK ½ cup pudding 4 ounces juice

LUNCH
¼ cup macaroni and
   cheese
2 orange slices
4 ounces whole milk
	SNACK
	½ bagel with cream
	   cheese
	4 ounces orange juice
		LUNCH
		¾ grilled-cheese
		   sandwich
		½ sliced tomato
		4 ounces whole milk

DINNER
2 tablespoons
   spaghetti with
   meatballs
1 teaspoon green
   beans
3 ounces whole milk
	LUNCH
	1 chicken drumstick
	1 plum
	6 ounces whole milk
		SNACK
		½ peach
		2 graham crackers
		2 ounces cranberry
		   juice

SNACK 4 ounces whole milk	SNACK 1 ounce cheese	DINNER ¾ cup spinach lasagna 4 ounces whole milk

	DINNER
	1 ounce ground
	   hamburger
	¼ cup garden peas
	½ cup mashed
	   potatoes
	4 ounces whole milk
		SNACK
		4 ounces whole milk
		1 chocolate cookie

	SNACK 8 ounces whole milk 1 gingerbread cookie	
Total calories: 598	Total calories: 1,660	Total calories: 1,402

AGES 3–10

Day 1: Low Calorie	*Day 2: High Calorie*	*Day 3: Average*
BREAKFAST 10 ounces orange juice	BREAKFAST Cheerios with 2 percent milk 4 ounces orange juice	BREAKFAST 2 slices French toast with syrup and butter 4 ounces grape juice
LUNCH 1 slice cheese pizza 8 ounces whole milk	LUNCH peanut butter and jelly sandwich 1 apple 8 ounces whole milk	LUNCH hotdog with bun ¾ cup french fries 8 ounces yogurt 8 ounces whole milk
SNACK single-serving bag of pretzels	SNACK banana frappé (6 ounces)	DINNER 2 ounces grilled fish ¾ cup new potatoes 1 cup coleslaw sourdough bread with margarine 6 ounces 2 percent milk
DINNER chicken pot pie (½ cup) 6 ounces 2 percent milk	DINNER cheeseburger salad with Russian dressing corn on the cob with butter slice of watermelon	
	SNACK 1½ cups popcorn with margarine 6 ounces orange juice	
Total calories: 1,050	Total calories: 2,335	Total calories: 1,728

AGES 10-18

Day 1: Low Calorie	Day 2: High Calorie	Day 3: Average
BREAKFAST blueberry pastry 8 ounces orange juice	BREAKFAST waffles topped with blueberries and syrup 8 ounces orange juice	BREAKFAST 2 scrambled eggs 2 slices whole wheat toast with margarine 4 ounces cran-grape juice
LUNCH slice of pepperoni pizza vanilla milk shake	LUNCH quiche salad with dressing 8 ounces skim milk	LUNCH 8 ounces yogurt turkey sandwich with provolone cheese
SNACK diet Coke	SNACK boysenberry yogurt frappé	SNACK single-serving bag of popcorn 12 ounces tonic
DINNER BBQ chicken breast ¾ cup asparagus ¾ cup pasta salad 8 ounces mineral water	DINNER grilled salmon steak red potatoes spinach salad with bacon dressing French bread	DINNER 4 ounces meatloaf ½ cup summer squash baked potato with margarine 8 ounces skim milk
SNACK 1 cup chocolate yogurt	SNACK Cheerios with skim milk	SNACK angel food cake with strawberries and whipped cream
Total calories: 1,850	Total calories: 2,400	Total calories: 2,175

over the course of a few days their total calorie intake averaged out to provide the energy and nutrients needed to stay healthy and grow along their normal curves.

Similar results came from studies done in the 1920s and 1930s by Canadian pediatrician Clara Davis, who also demonstrated that children get enough to eat when nutritious food is made available to them.

Still more recently, a study done between 1986 and 1989 headed by Steven Shea, M.D., of Columbia University College of Physicians and Surgeons, and published in *Pediatrics* in 1992 (Volume 90, No. 4), showed that *in their everyday environment* young children will self-regulate their energy consumption over the course of a day.

Parents who worry about how their child eats can be reassured by these studies. A child may appear to eat "like a bird" or "like a horse," but when offered a variety of nutritious foods, most of them obtain the nutrition they need for growth, without being coerced by parents to eat in any given amount. While they won't always make the right food choices—as many of the candy companies would have you believe they would—they will choose nutritious foods if they are educated about how it helps them grow—and are given access to healthy foods.

This, then, is the parent's role—*to educate children about healthy food choices, and to give them ready access to good nutrition.*

Monotonous Food Choices
Go with the Territory

A varied diet is the ideal, but as anyone who has ever dealt with toddlers or young children knows, they don't care one bit what you think about a varied diet; they latch onto one food for breakfast, lunch, and dinner and that's the only thing they want to eat.

At age two, Josh would only eat a scrambled egg at dinner. Scrambled egg, catsup, and juice—that was his dinner every night until he was about three and a half years old. It appeared that eggs were all he ate, but in fact, during the rest of the day he had other things—hot cereal in the morning (he loved farina); a peanut butter and jelly sandwich for lunch; and snacks including cookies, milk, various cheeses, potato chips, pretzels, and popcorn.

In other words, Josh managed to have quite a wide variety of foods in his diet, but it was that one egg every night for dinner that caught everybody's attention and even caused some concern—one neighbor even worried Josh would "get heart disease" from eating all those eggs. However, from a nutritional standpoint, there was nothing wrong with it. An egg is an excellent source of high-quality nutrition, containing approximately 15 percent of the RDA for protein, riboflavin, and folate; 30 percent of the RDA for vitamin B_{12} and phosphorus, and in lesser amounts, iron and zinc. As for heart disease, clogged arteries were extremely unlikely at Josh's age, as was the risk of the eggs causing a buildup of cholesterol in the body (for more on cholesterol, see Chapter 2).

Josh's monotonous preference for an egg every night for dinner went along very consistently with his stage of development and was no different from the food preferences of other children his age—children whose "mono-food desires" eventually peter out or, one day, abruptly stop when the child "does not like" those foods anymore!

Today, at age eight, Josh eats eggs about twice a month ("scrambled loose with catsup") if he feels like it. That's his choice—no one tells him he should or should not eat them.

Avoiding the Notion of Nutritional "Slip-Ups"

Instead of worrying about a child's erratic eating, many parents would do better resolving the issue *they* have with erratic feeding.

Often parents will blame themselves for being erratic or inconsistent with feeding their children meals. Perhaps out of guilt for having a career that takes them away from their children, or because their own poor eating habits cause guilt, one day they will allow a trip to the local fast-food restaurant and the next, outlaw that same kind of food. Or they "slip up"—for example, they are out on the soccer or baseball field with their child, close to lunchtime, and an ice cream truck rolls by. That presents a quandary. Is it all right to skip lunch and have ice cream instead? Is a child's nutrition ruined by this approach? Some mothers and fathers will stop the ice cream truck, place their order, and think "Oh, dear, I am giving my child an ice cream cone instead of a good lunch. I feel terrible." Or they will run out of milk, make a quick trip to the supermarket, find that the supply of low-fat milk is gone, buy a container of whole milk, and then feel terrible.

These "slip-ups" are fine and could be redefined as normal variations or viable options. No child is going to die from a glass of whole milk, and ice cream for lunch under the circumstances described confirms that a parent's priorities are in order—participating with the child and the child's teammates outdoors instead of cutting the fun short for a conventional lunch.

HINTS AND TIPS FOR CONFLICT-FREE MEALS

By working with the "natural appetite" theory rather than against it, you can avoid making an issue out of meals today at the same time that you help your child avoid making food a problem later on.

- Envision your child as a "natural eater." The natural eater is not picky because he or she eats when cued by hunger.
- Consider that you have the responsibility for supplying nutritious foods; your child has the responsibility for how much of those foods to eat.
- Do not be surprised if children ask for food every two or three hours. Listen when they say they are hungry and give them something to eat.
- Provide ready access to nutritious snacks, which are an essential part of a child's natural eating pattern and diet. (For more on snacks and snacking, see Chapter 2.)
- Do not expect mealtime to be "quality time" with your child. For many busy families today, the time spent together relaxing after meals can be more enjoyable than the time spent together during meals.
- Always serve food to children in small amounts. Better yet, encourage children to serve their own helpings and to ask for seconds if they want them. Many children are intimidated by large portions of food on their plate.
- Approach meals by accepting that no particular food has to be eaten at any one meal, and no complete meal that's put out has to be eaten. Instead, have your child "try a small bite" of what he or she doesn't want, and leave it at that.
- Give nutritious foods top priority. Make a variety of good foods available for children to choose from.
- Keep offering new foods even if they are rejected. "In general, children prefer familiar foods and are reluctant to try strange ones," explains Dr. Birch. In her studies, she found that a child might need to be encouraged to taste a new food as many as ten times before that food would be deemed familiar enough to be accepted.
- Do not make food part of a reward system. Offer food with no strings attached.
- Encourage children to have a taste of whatever is on their

plate, but give dessert equal billing in a meal regardless of what gets eaten first.

- Promote self-feeding. Children can master feeding skills by age two; let them feed themselves.
- Don't hover. You can help with table manners, but standing (or sitting) watch over a child's intake of food promotes indigestion for everyone.
- Let the growth chart tell the story. Most parents form their impression of their children's appetite at mealtimes from what they see but because they are not around during much of the day, this assessment is only based on a very small portion of the day.
- If you are concerned with your child's food intake or appetite, discuss it with your pediatrician. Parents who are not convinced of their child's healthy progress can do a diet diary to get a sense of what a child is eating, provided they do not become obsessed with it. Or compare what your child eats over a few days with the foods that are suggested in the chart on page 109. Remember the bottom line: what the growth charts show.
- Read on for special considerations relating to individual meals—breakfast, lunch, and dinner.

Mealtime Food Phrases
Parents Should Avoid

"Save your appetite for later."
"But I cooked it just for you!"
"Is that *all* you're going to eat?"
"Finish what's on your plate."
"If you want dessert, eat all of your dinner."
"That's enough for now; you've had enough to eat."

Is a "Good Breakfast" Essential?

There is a whole body of research that has attempted to determine whether giving a child a "good breakfast"—one that delivers a third of the energy requirements for the day—would have a beneficial effect on intellectual performance, social interactions, and energy levels at school. It was hoped that there would be a clear correlation between a highly nutritious breakfast and children who were happier, more energetic, and more productive in school than those who had little or no breakfast. In fact, the studies showed that some children did better on calculating problems with no breakfast, while others who had a good breakfast did better on short-term memory problems.

Does this mean your child should skip breakfast if he or she has math first thing in the morning, or should have a good breakfast if he or she starts out with reading comprehension? Of course not. What it demonstrates is that food in the morning is not the whole story in determining a child's ability to succeed at school or in meeting his or her nutrition needs. Breakfast is an excellent opportunity for children to eat a significant portion of their daily nutritional requirements, and youngsters who eat breakfast at home tend to have a better nutritional intake over the course of a day. Some children prefer a small breakfast (a bowl of cereal with milk is very nutritious) and some of them can even skip breakfast with no ill effect. In our view, *if a child can get the energy and nutrients he or she needs over the course of a day, there is no need to hold breakfast to any one nutrition standard.* This approach allows room for individual eating patterns and food preferences, while providing flexibility for resolving conflicts that arise over breakfast.

Easy Breakfast Guidelines

Recognize Your Child's Individual Food Needs in the Morning.
As a parent, you need to get some sense of what your young-ster's energy requirements are for the morning. With some children, hunger can affect performance. If a report from a teacher informed you that your child was doing poorly in school, an important first determination would be whether or not that child had ready access to food throughout the day. If he or she goes to a school that provides snack machines in the hallway and the opportunity to get a snack during a morning break between classes, then it makes no difference whether the child eats breakfast at home or not. However, if you know your child will become very hungry an hour or so after skip-ping breakfast at home, has no access to food between classes, and will be listless and tired until he or she eats lunch, you should encourage the child to eat some food at home or on the way to school. Get him or her out of bed fifteen minutes earlier for breakfast; or give the child options for eating as he or she dresses or walks or rides to school (a bagel and a juice to go).

Think of Breakfast Foods As Anything a Child Is Comfortable Eating. An advantage in having the typical American breakfast of orange juice and cereal with milk is that it provides the opportunity for receiving some vitamin C (in juice); carbohy-drates, protein, and fiber (in cereal); calcium and other miner-als, protein, and vitamin D (in milk). However, if you view the day's intake of nutrients in a circle rather than in a straight line, breakfast becomes only one point on that circle. While we are all for the first foods of the day being nutritious, no food is unacceptable or harmful in the morning, and there is no particular way to eat it. Breakfast could be anything from a bowl of cereal and milk or microwave waffles topped with fruit and jam; a container of yogurt while getting dressed; a glass of juice at home and a bagel eaten on the walk to school; a scrambled egg in a whole wheat pita pocket—or it could be leftover Chinese food or pizza. From a nutritional standpoint, all of these would be fine food choices.

We are willing to push this idea even further and say that while a can of soda with a corn muffin might not qualify as a "good breakfast," if breakfast is one link on the food chain for the day, then there is probably nothing wrong with a child's request for soda as part of breakfast—although we cannot recommend canned soda as a major beverage for anyone. If a child had soda all day and nothing else to drink, that would be different; but if that same child at lunch had chocolate milk with a sandwich, apple juice in the afternoon with a snack, and plain low-fat milk at dinner, then it really doesn't matter if he or she had the soda instead of milk or juice at breakfast, and the milk or juice rather than the soda at lunch. Looking at soda within the day's context, it provides 110 calories of sugar, a corn muffin provides carbohydrates and other nutrients, and from an energy standpoint, they add up to roughly a 300-calorie breakfast, albeit one lacking in many of the nutrients necessary for optimal growth and development.

If You Find Yourself Fighting over Breakfast, Ask Yourself Whether Food Is Really the Issue. One mother got into a major fight with her twelve-year-old daughter every morning, insisting that unless she ate a full breakfast at home before she went to school, the daughter would not do well in school. The daughter would have none of it—she always ran late and barely made the school bus every day.

As it turned out, the fighting over food was just one of many other fights this mother and daughter were having; the daughter wanted more autonomy and the mother was using nutritional rules to exercise control. In fact, the daughter was growing well and doing just fine in school.

We were able to help them reach a compromise. By mutual agreement, the daughter would have the breakfast foods of her choice—a container of juice and a buttered bagel—on the school bus. The mother would forget about the eggs and toast and juice and sit-down breakfast at home; her role would be to make the bagels and juice available as her child went out the door.

As this example illustrates, the ability to "let go" in areas that are trivial or meaningless—particularly when it involves a child's changing developmental stages—is a valuable skill in parenting (for more on teen transitions, see page 186).

Positive Lunchbox Strategies

If you are one of the many parents today who packs up a lunchbox of healthy foods for your child to eat at school, a visit to your child's classroom at noon would quickly dispel any preconceived view of how that lunch goes down. Most youngsters will dive for the cookies first, eat a bite or two out of the sandwich and the apple, throw away the rest, and turn to the serious business at hand—trading to get the candy bar or cupcake that has been unpacked by the classmate next to them.

For many children, lunch at school or preschool is their first exposure to making their own food choices. Parents are not there to monitor what goes down, teachers are not going to chide their students for what they do or do not eat, peer acceptance is often going to determine what a child will (or won't) eat.

Giving children choices for lunch is the first step to having them eat what's packed; when they are old enough, they can pack their own lunch foods:

- Seven-year-old Abe usually gets an apple juice pack, a tuna fish and mayo sandwich on white bread, an apple, two or three cookies, and a favorite candy bar.
- Nine-year-old James has announced he's off peanut butter and jelly sandwiches and wants a salami sandwich with lettuce in his lunchbox—that's what his friend Matt had for lunch yesterday. A thermos of chocolate milk, a bunch

of grapes, and a piece of homemade carrot cake round off lunch for the day.

- Twelve-year-old Sally "brown bags" lunch herself: a container of strawberry-banana yogurt, half a cinnamon-raisin bagel with butter, an apple, and a few chocolate chip cookies. (She alternates this with her own vegetable-pasta salad, a "pita pack" of salad greens, and Middle Eastern food, all prepared and chilled the night before.)
- Fifteen-year-old Emily also packs her own lunch: a ham or turkey sandwich, a bottle of soda, some carrots or cucumbers, a pile of cookies, and some crackers for a snack later on—all in what appears to be a fifty-pound sack she carries out of the house every morning.
- Seventeen-year-old Adam—Who knows what he eats? He buys his own lunch and from all appearances, he's doing just fine.

As you can see, this varied approach caters to the individual preferences of children and reflects their stage of development. Once again, whether you fix your children's lunch or they fix their own, they deserve an active role in choosing what to pack.

PACKING POINTERS

- Solicit lunch requests or make healthful suggestions for lunch; let them know that you are open to the foods they want.
- Honor all requests. Children will be less inclined to trade for foods if they get what they want.
- Aim to please. If your child comes home and tells you that on a scale of one to ten the lunch you packed was a zero, discuss ways to improve it. Avoid foods that other kids will think are weird.
- Use lunch foods to help promote good nutrition. We don't make a distinction between "health food" and "junk

food"; the real issue has to do with how much nutrition is in each particular food. Obviously, some foods are more nutritious than others, bite for bite, and it is variety that ensures good nutrition. There's nothing wrong with a high-fat salami sandwich one day if on other days it alternates with a low-fat choice like turkey or tuna.
• For the child who packs his or her own lunch, or buys food in school, give some guidelines for including nutritious foods.

The parent who points out that a piece of fruit is a good idea to take to school each day is a good parent, whereas the parent who says nothing about fruit as his or her child packs candy bars and potato chips every day is not doing the child any favors.

If there is a choice about ordering what to drink at school, leave the choice up to the child. Chocolate milk, apple juice, 1 percent milk, 2 percent milk, or even whole milk as a drink at eleven o'clock in the morning on a school day would be fine, as would a candy bar for a snack or part of lunch, provided the child is also encouraged to have a piece of fruit sometimes for a snack. Balance in the diet is the key, evaluating food choices over the course of several days and not just one.

The Ritual of Dinner, Revised

In most families today, it takes some effort to time dinner so everyone eats together, and it takes even more effort to make that time enjoyable. Waiting for everyone to get home, insisting on good manners, good eating habits, and good conversation—that's a lot to expect when people are usually strung out, tired, and cranky.

If you feel pressured to live up to the ideal of the "family dinner," then the concept of dinner should be revised. There are better ways for families to come together and relax in the evening.

TIPS FOR DESTRESSING DINNERTIME

- Look at dinner as one opportunity for everybody being together, but not the only opportunity. Shift the focus from the family dinner to the family, and find new ways to enjoy a relaxed time together.
- Feed children first if they are hungry; they can join you at the table later while you eat. It's much better to give a hungry child an early supper if it makes him or her more relaxed with you later on.
- Use the kitchen as the evening gathering place—for food, conversation, and evening work. If you come home after everyone else has eaten dinner, invite your child to join you while you eat. The child can finish off his or her homework; you can proofread an essay.
- Every now and then, set aside Saturday or Sunday afternoon for an early family dinner.
- Make a special occasion out of going out together for lunch or dinner, or ordering in.
- When you do eat together, shift the focus from the food and how much is eaten to a more enjoyable subject.
- Make available a nutritious alternative to the food served at dinnertime, for example, juice and a peanut butter and jelly sandwich, or a bowl of cereal, fruit, and milk. Encourage the child who chooses not to eat what's served to prepare their own alternative.

12

◆ ◆ ◆ ◆

Resolving the "Junk Food" Dilemma

You can avoid a big area of aggravation and conflict by accepting that when given a choice, children will often choose foods that many adults classify as "unhealthy." *Provided these foods are not fully replacing a child's regular diet,* we say there is nothing wrong with children choosing them.

Outlawing certain foods may even be detrimental. If children are always told that "good" foods are "all-natural" and "bad" foods are manufactured, processed, or contain artificial ingredients, they will begin to feel guilty about exploring different tastes—especially those sweet, salty, buttery tastes that are universally appealing and often found in the category that is referred to as "junk food."

What Is Junk Food?

The term *junk food* has several connotations, all of them negative. Some people perceive it as food that is so highly processed it has no nutritional value and thus contains "empty" calories. Others view it as containing too much of one ingredient, such as fat or salt or sugar, or too many artificial ingredients, thus making it harmful.

Depending on interpretation, many different foods are thus categorized as "junk foods"—from hot dogs and TV dinners, to packaged snacks and candy bars, to potato chips and chocolate milk.

Casting foods as "junk"—just as casting them as "bad"—has little nutritional significance. From a nutritional standpoint, *any* food that is eaten to the exclusion of all else for weeks at a time can eventually cause malnourishment—be it lettuce or carrots, candy or canned soda. Of course, this rarely happens. Someone would have to be locked in a room with a steady diet of candy bars or lettuce leaves for days and days for problems to occur.

In keeping with the guidelines set forth by the American Dietetic Association and the American Academy of Pediatrics—that for healthy individuals who are not for medical reasons on a restriced diet, there is no one food that is bad and no food that should be on the forbidden list—we urge parents to go easy on casting certain foods in a negative light, or qualifying them as "junk."

From a medical standpoint, if a child is eating a variety of foods, growing on his or her curve, and developing well, that child can have any food he or she wants.

Conflicts with Grandparents and Caregivers

The issue of snack foods, "junk foods," and treats often comes up with grandparents and older caregivers who, because of their life-style, approach food and eating quite differently from many parents today.

Most grandparents today were raised in times when there were very few food rules for anyone, and little knowledge about the health risks that have created those rules. Those who are old enough to have lived through the Depression and Second World War experienced food shortages and other hardships that gave them a special appreciation for rich foods, treat foods, and large amounts of food—an appreciation they see nothing wrong with sharing with their children and grandchildren.

The different perspectives of generations on food as well as other everyday issues such as money, where to live, where to eat Thanksgiving dinner, and how to raise the children can create an atmosphere of tension *that should not involve children*. If the child is caught between the standards of two generations—not wanting to disappoint the grandparent by refusing a treat, and not wanting to disappoint the parent by eating a food he or she doesn't have at home—the conflict and guilt that child feels is going be more harmful than any nutritional disadvantage from eating the food. To avoid this, whether or not caregivers or grandparents give children certain snacks or treats, the child's needs must come first: *There should be no mixed messages conveyed to the child that might make him or her feel guilty.*

When both generations are willing to meet this objective, grandparents and parents can find ways to eliminate the conflict, either by conceding to the person whose feelings are strongest, for or against the treat; or by working out a compromise that will not detract from the child's enjoyment.

If a compromise cannot be negotiated, outside advice should be solicited, starting with the child's pediatrician.

In the case of nonfamily caregivers, unless the child is gaining weight too rapidly, as shown on the growth chart or in the educated opinion of the pediatrician, parents should not outlaw certain foods but instead suggest broad categories from which the child can choose—fruits, vegetables, ice cream of choice, chocolate candies, etc.

Popular Snack Foods:
How Much Is Too Much?

Without recommending or endorsing them, here are guidelines for what we would consider reasonable amounts of certain popular foods that a child might choose if no one else were around.

Candy Bars A child who has three to five candy bars a week is nobody's problem; one who has one or two candy bars a day may be nobody's problem either, if he or she is also eating a variety of other, more nutritious foods.

On the other hand, four to five candy bars a day would be excessive, and it would be wrong if the child who had two or more candy bars were also running out of the house before breakfast, and were not hungry at lunch and dinner because he or she was filling up on snack foods and candy instead. A heavy reliance on candy bars and snack foods indicates a pretty unbalanced diet.

As for choosing what type of candy and candy bars is reasonable, the primary consideration is whether the choice is age appropriate, that is, whether or not by eating it, the child runs the risk of choking. In that light, M&M's would not be an appropriate choice for a two-year-old, whereas for an older child they might be fine. The hardness of a candy bar is another important consideration—whether or not a child might break a tooth biting into a very hard, thick chocolate bar or something else.

As for content, bowing to public pressure, candy manufacturers have come up with candy bars that are more nutritionally balanced than they were in the past, many of them containing a decreased amount of saturated fat, and starches instead of pure sugar. Check the labels for ingredients. Candy bars containing coconut or cashew nuts, which are both very high in saturated fat, should be eaten in moderation. That is, if you saw that your child was only buying coconut candy bars, five a week, that would be a reason to steer him or her to something else.

Chewing Gum Sugarless gum is not a problem; nonnutritive sweeteners do not cause cancer. There is no nutritional or safety issue with sugarless gum or for any gum, and it would only be a dental issue if the child were chewing gum all the time and neglecting to brush his or her teeth. (The use of fluoride has drastically cut down on tooth decay, making this not nearly the issue it was for children in the past.)

Soda There's nothing "bad" about soda, which is essentially bubble water and flavoring; on the other hand, an average soda contains roughly ten teaspoons of sugar, and the carbonation fills the stomach up with gas rather than with nutrients. Sodas (and this includes diet soda) do not contain vitamins or protein.

For these reasons, once again we cannot recommend soda as a regular drink for anyone, particularly a growing child who needs a variety of nutrients along with calories. And yet one needs to be realistic. If your child goes for pizza with friends, of course he or she can have a soda, just like everyone else. If the child wants to have a soda while doing homework, fine; a can of soda a day is no problem. On the other hand, there are some drinks that should be drunk less frequently than others, and soda should be considered one of them. Nutritious drinks should also be available, as drinks are one good, fast way for children to obtain nutrients.

Diet Soda No one is going to die or have hallucinations or develop bladder cancer from having sodas that contain artificial sweeteners, and if a child prefers to have a diet soda instead of one with sugar, that's fine. However, unless the child is diabetic, there is no advantage to having diet soda, certainly not for weight control. Artificially sweetened sodas and diet beverages satisfy the perception that they help to cut down on calories, but people who drink a fair amount of them tend to make up for the calories elsewhere in their diet.

Salty Foods Foods such as potato chips, corn chips, and cheese twists usually contain a high amount of fat—that, and not the salt, is what to watch. When alternated with other foods, and without exceeding guidelines for fat (approximately 30 percent of total calories a day) we have no problem with a child's having these foods.

Peanut Butter Fat content is one of the reasons that peanut butter doesn't get on everybody's list of good foods. Up until recently, most commercial peanut butter was emulsified with a saturated fat to help make it smooth and creamy. Due to consumer pressure, most peanut butter manufacturers no longer add saturated fat to peanut butter. If your child wants a peanut butter and jelly sandwich at lunch every day, that's a very good combination of nutrients. With chocolate milk? Great. No problem. For children who are eating a varied diet, we can't think of a single food that has to be very closely monitored for better health—provided it does not crowd out other foods.

TIPS FOR RESOLVING CONFLICTS OVER "JUNK" FOODS AND SNACK FOODS

- Avoid outlawing any particular snack food. Keep a variety of foods on hand and let children make their own snack choices from them.
- Include snack foods as part of the "five-a-day" fruit and vegetable guideline (see page 120), the goal of which is to encourage eating more nutritious foods at the expense of highly saturated, or fatty foods.
- Do not make children feel guilty for wanting "junk food" for snacks. Let them have it as part of a variety of other snacks that are more nutritious.

- If your child asks for a snack close to dinnertime, do not tell him or her, "It will ruin your appetite." Give the child "meal foods"—cheese, raw vegetables, etc.—instead.
- Avoid setting snacking limits. Judge amounts by personal experience with your own child. If two or three ounces of chips in the afternoon keeps him or her going until lunch or dinner, that's fine. Active children who eat halfway decent, balanced meals can snack all they want.
- Avoid negotiating for limits—for example, saying if your child has chocolate milk in school for a snack, he or she cannot have it at home.
- Go back to the growth charts if snacking seems excessive. If growth is in the normal range, leave the child alone.

Fight Scenes—Rating Your Attitude

Check off what best describes your reaction in the following six scenarios.

1. You've just formed a toddler play group. All the other mothers but you insist on toddler snacks and juices from the health food store. Do you:
   a. consider dropping out of the play group;
   b. prefer a range of snacks but say nothing, thinking your food standards for your child are probably too low;
   c. propose that snacks be supplied individually, and suggest that the other mothers buy a copy of this book?

2. Your toddler in the supermarket wants a box of sugar-coated, Day-Glo Dinosaur Cereal; you want to buy something "more nutritious." Do you:
   a. put the cereal back on the shelf and ignore your child's protests;
   b. put it in the cart and deposit it behind the boxes of dried cat food in the next aisle;
   c. buy both cereals and trade off casually?

3. Your child's grandmother brings candy every time she visits. Do you:

   a. refuse to allow the candy in your house;

   b. intercept the gift and put it away for "later";

   c. check to see that it is age-appropriate (i.e., of a size that will not cause choking and a texture that won't cause broken teeth), and let the child have it?

4. It's Halloween. Do you:

   a. keep your child from trick-or-treating with friends because the event centers on candy;

   b. take the candy out of your child's trick-or-treat bag and only leave in fruit and nut treats;

   c. follow your child's inclinations, check the candy for being age appropriate, and let him or her decide what to eat over time?

5. The teacher has told your second grader's class that "only nutritious snacks" should be brought in to school. Do you:

   a. give your child a bag of carrot sticks to share with her friends;

   b. call around to see what other parents have brought in to school so you can use the information to negotiate with your child;

   c. write a note for the teacher the day before the birthday to say that your son will be sending in his choice for birthday snack the next day—cupcakes he wants to share with the class?

6. Your thirteen-year-old daughter, who has a chocolate bar every day on the way home from school with her friends, is concerned because her skin is breaking out. Do you:

   a. tell her the candy is causing her skin to break out and she should not have it;

   b. try to make her feel better by telling her she shouldn't worry about pimples—everyone her age has them;

   c. say nothing about the candy but suggest ways she can help clear up the blemishes, for example, by washing her face well and keeping it free from oil and makeup, by eating a balanced diet, and by getting enough sleep?

7. Your sixteen-year-old son has just left the dinner table, once again refusing to eat his salad (or spinach). Do you:
   a. yell at him to get back to the table and eat his greens, telling him he won't be able to join his friends for their nightly basketball game if he doesn't;
   b. turn to his younger brother or sister and tell *him* or *her* it's unhealthy not to eat vegetables;
   c. let him go and enjoy your salad; continue serving greens at dinnertime, and also provide fruits and vegetables that on-the-run members of the family can choose for snacks?

Self-evaluation:

a = try to be more relaxed about food issues, and probably in other areas involving control over your child.

b = you are ambivalent about certain foods and food issues, potentially in conflict. To gain more confidence, turn to the chapters in this book that relate to children's growth, or to areas that concern you.

c = keep up the good work.

13

❖　❖　❖　❖

Food Tensions
at Transition Stages

Tensions between parents and children over food and other issues can arise off and on throughout childhood but they are most likely to occur during the transitional stages of childhood. In this chapter, we look at three of these stages—the newborn arriving into the world, the baby becoming a toddler, the child moving into puberty and adolescence—explaining why these particular times can add a special layer of stress to the parent-child relationship, and what to do about it.

The Newborn
and the Postpartum Adjustment

The first weeks home from the hospital with a newborn can be very stressful—as one set of new parents said, "Now how do we keep him alive?"

Newborn babies cry to communicate their needs; that's all they can do. Some of those needs are urgent—food, warmth, survival—but babies also cry for many other reasons, some of them inexplicable. Questions about feeding inevitably arise. Is she hungry? Is he getting enough food? Is she *still* hungry? Does he have indigestion? Colic? Something else?

The guidelines given for feeding a baby in Chapter 9 can help new parents determine whether the baby is getting enough food; here we focus on the tensions that accompany the arrival of a newborn.

The Mother-Baby Relationship Mothers and their babies should be essentially happy in their relationship. Babies learn through generous care and a ready supply of food that they are valued, that their inner feelings can be communicated, first through tears, then through looks and pointing, and finally through words. Through the responses to these communications, they discover that their needs can be met—that there is someone out there who loves them and, as D. W. Winnicott, the English pediatrician and child psychiatrist, stated, "that something can be done about something." (Children who are neglected at this age feel the opposite—that they are not valued and that nothing can be done about anything.)

In feeding a baby, then, mothers should feel that they're doing what is right for their baby. If the baby is not happy or the mother feels she's not doing the right thing, that's a serious concern because it is going to affect how the mother attaches to that baby—how close they can get, how happy the baby is going to be, how good the mother is going to feel about herself. Disappointment on any of these counts can set up a pattern of behavior that can have quite serious consequences throughout childhood and into adult life. If baby or mother is not happy, that is in and of itself a concern that easily gets translated into thoughts, behaviors, and struggles about food.

Clearly a mother who's unhappy about not being able to breast-feed, for whatever the reason, is a much bigger problem in terms of the baby's development than a mother who has freely made her choice. Or a mother who cannot hold her baby either for her own psychological reasons (for example, depression) or because she's being overworked—that's also a much bigger problem in terms of attachment than whether you use breast milk or formula.

Sometimes societal pressures interfere when a mother is stressed by standards set by her own personal and cultural background. Whatever the perception, the baby's appearance tells the world the mother is a good mother, that she knows how to feed and take care of her baby. As the need to measure up to these standards can lead to problems with how a mother attaches to her baby, resulting from unmet expectations, it is important that mothers be relieved of the thought that they have to show the world their baby is well fed or else risk being thought of as doing a bad job parenting.

If the baby's not happy or the mother's not happy, that is reason enough to get help—the earlier the better.

"Goodness of Fit" Babies normally cry when they are hungry, and one the most rewarding things about feeding a young infant is picking the infant up, feeding him or her, and having the baby coo back at you and rest happily in your arms after finishing feeding. Normal, healthy babies can also cry for no identifiable reason—a pattern that typically increases and peaks at about six to eight weeks—and a crying baby can make any person, especially a mother, feel frustrated, guilty, or inadequate if she cannot console the baby.

In their book, *Temperament and Behavior Disorders in Children,* child psychiatrists Stella Chess and Alexander Thomas use the term *goodness of fit* in evaluating how smoothly a mother's temperament or personality meshes with her baby's needs, how well she adapts to them psychologically.

Goodness of fit—or lack of it—is one of the underpinnings of the discomfort that some mothers can have with their baby due to difficulties attaching. It's not that these parents are abnormal or disturbed, they are just more sensitive to crying and would not do well with a baby who cries a lot. Or they need a regular schedule themselves and will have problems with a baby who demands food at erratic intervals. If that is the case, their discomfort may get translated into anxiety about food or control issues about food when in fact that is not really the issue. For example, their response to a baby who gets hungry unexpectedly after two hours instead of four might be to continue firmly to hold to a rigid feeding schedule—the more the baby cries, the more the mother digs in and waits. Whether because of her priorities or her personality, this can turn into a miserable, vicious cycle in which the mother, in feeling more like a failure, tries even harder to stick to the rules that she's read somewhere; and the baby, in not being comforted, becomes even more miserable. In fact, what would probably break the cycle for this particular mother and for her baby is more food, a different schedule, more nurturing and holding, help at home, transferring the baby from breast to bottle, and reconsidering work issues.

Colicky Babies Any baby who appears to be crying more often than usual in between feedings, or who is awake most of the time crying, or awake often throughout the night and crying, even to the third or fourth week of life should be discussed with your pediatrician to review the baby's health, evaluate the crying episodes, and have the baby examined to be sure his or her health is fine. The problem may be treatable or it may simply be colic, which is defined as increased crying time during the first few months of life.

Colic is a very common problem, and occurs in healthy babies who are growing, feeding very nicely, and falling asleep after they finish feeding—but then wake up very quickly after that and cry inconsolably.

Unfortunately, there is no clear cause for colic. Rarely, or occasionally, it is due to allergy, but that is quite the exception. However, we mention allergy here because in the last few years, as a result of carefully conducted research, it has become clear that a small minority of infants with persistent colic may be allergic to cow's milk proteins, which are found in standard infant formulas. In these studies, with the use of placebo-controlled trials to establish the diagnosis of milk allergy, the colic disappeared when these same infants were placed on a hypoallergenic infant formula. Over time, however, the benefit of feeding a hypoallergenic formula seemed to diminish.

In the case of diagnosing milk allergy, it is important to recognize that colic is rarely, if ever, the only symptom. Other symptoms include vomiting, diarrhea, wheezing, and rashes. Moreover, in 90 percent or more of infants with colic, milk allergy is not the cause of crying.

If you have a colicky baby and you and your pediatrician rule out milk allergy, there remains nothing to do but to try to comfort the baby while the colic lasts (see below). At the same time, it is critical for parents and other caregivers to allow for "break time" from such babies and to try to look ahead to the time when those difficult crying times will gradually diminish (and they will). In the meantime, once again, it is not unusual for babies to be perfectly healthy, well nourished, and satisfied after they finish feeding—and still cry a lot.

Difficult Babies—Even More of a Challenge Most babies have different styles and different needs, which can be evident right from the first weeks of life, even before parents have had much influence on personality development. Some babies can be very hard to read. Some of them will scream all the time and never seem satisfied even after being fed. They will be hard to calm down, unable to soothe themselves, never establish a feeding schedule and they'll get upset more readily and more intensely. It's hard to say why it is—perhaps because their nervous systems are not as mature as other babies', or perhaps because they are showing some of the personality traits of their parents—but that's just the way it is, the way they're built, the way they are wired. In any case, while they are not necessarily going to grow up abnormal (although Chess and

Thomas's work suggests these babies are at higher risk for emotional problems), these babies are not easy to live with and they are not easy to attach to because they need a different style of interaction than do other babies. They need parents who are flexible and able to make special efforts to try to adapt to their particular needs. They demand more attention, patience, and empathy. Sometimes this involves holding the baby more, feeding the baby more, giving him or her a pacifier, changing the diaper more, taking long stroller walks, or simplifying the baby's schedule. Because these babies' own neurological organization does not permit them to calm easily, external factors such as being held, or being given a pacifier or more feedings can make an enormous difference in calming them down—as can some of the suggestions in the section that follows.

Soothing a Crying or Difficult Baby Some physicians and psychologists suggest that you let babies cry right through their crying time so they can learn to console themselves; but we come down on the side of responding to that baby's cries— especially in the first month.

Babies are people and, in our view, people have a couple of key issues that develop during infancy. One is the sense of self-esteem—the feeling that you are worth something. It is hard to imagine that the baby who is crying alone, especially in the first few months of life, feels very valued. This baby certainly cannot understand the world and is very limited in his or her ability to self-comfort. He or she feels quite alone and isolated. As with any person who is crying, the baby likes to be comforted and likes company. A baby certainly does value loving attention, despite the fact that he or she may continue to cry, or appear to be inconsolable. Surely the baby needs that feeling that if I'm crying, I can be fed. If I'm cold, I can be warmed. If I am wet, I can be changed. If I need to be held, I can be held. In terms of basic personality traits, to feel that you are valued and to feel that something can be done to relieve your suffering are two very positive attributes that are well worth encouraging and fostering in a personality at a very young age.

Physical Contact As a Means of Comfort Holding babies has been shown to be beneficial to both mother and baby, especially with babies who cry a lot. It can improve their disposition. This was demonstrated in a study published in 1991 in a journal of the American Academy of Pediatrics, involving ninety-nine infants and mothers at the Montreal Children's Hospital Research Institute. Some of the mothers were asked to hold their babies or carry them in a carrier for at least three hours a day. Diary entries reporting on their babies' behavior indicated that those infants who were carried more often than previously cried 43 percent less than they had in a twenty-four-hour period before, and 51 percent less during the evening hours when measured at six weeks, the age of peak crying. Similar but smaller decreases were found four, eight, and twelve weeks after birth. "The relative lack of carrying in our society may predispose normal infants to crying and colic," the researchers stated.

However, a comparison of the style with which babies are handled in various cultures, past and present, shows how well they adapt—from being kept constantly next to their mother for warmth and mobility, to becoming involved in physical contact for only a few hours at a time and, in either case, turning out just fine.

Pacifiers Pacifiers provide suckling without nutrition. Are pacifiers habit forming? Do they cause a baby's teeth to come in crooked? Do they lead to obesity? Many parents are concerned that pacifiers are a problem, but in fact, for those infants who will take them, they not only improve the baby's swallowing and sucking coordination, but may even improve the baby's ability to move food down the digestive tract and develop more mature patterns of intestinal movement.

There is no harm in giving a pacifier, particularly if it can help soothe the infant. If a baby needs to suck as a means of self-comforting, and the mother is using the pacifier as a part of her total care, then the pacifier will make the baby feel that some of his or her suffering or inner feelings can be soothed. As a result we're teaching the baby two things: (1) that he or she is valued and loved, and (2) that something can be done when something is wrong.

On the negative side, and back to the notion of a baby's self-esteem, if a mother is giving a child a pacifier as a way of keeping the child quiet or using a pacifier selfishly for her own need to avoid contact with the baby, then that's the beginning of a pattern that's going to undervalue or devalue the child. The baby left alone may temporarily feel better having a pacifier, but the pacifier will not satisfy the baby's need for contact.

HINTS FOR SOOTHING A CRYING BABY

- Pick up and hold the baby.
- Offer a pacifier.
- Change the diaper.
- Adjust clothing and temperature—warmer or cooler.
- Hold and rock the baby rhythmically.
- Turn on music or a music box.
- Check the baby's feeding schedule; he or she may need more food.
- Take the baby out for a drive.
- Carry the baby in a baby carrier against your body; walk outdoors.
- Visit a playground or school yard. (Let the baby hear other children.)
- Visit a friend.
- Take turns soothing the baby with someone else, but stay with that baby.

- Get help and advice; share your concerns.
- Call your pediatrician if crying is persistent.

Baby to Toddler:
The High-Chair Adventure

Control issues typically accompany the transition of a baby into toddlerhood.

Eating in a high chair rather than on someone's lap symbolizes that another stage is under way—the baby is beginning to have a separate identity from the parent. It is a delicate time. The parents' sense of satisfaction in watching their baby's very definite personality emerge is at the same time a bittersweet loss—of the baby who will no longer accept the cuddling, feeding, and other activities that were taken for granted before six months of age. Eating, which requires sitting still, interferes with the movement of the toddler who is just beginning to walk and express him- or herself, however contrarily, in gestures and words.

Tensions unique to this time very definitely involve food and the toddler's need to practice his or her "self-feeding" skills. Controlling the baby's food—insisting on feeding him or her—may be a parent's way of delaying this earliest manifestation of the baby's emerging self. On the other hand, introducing real foods and establishing self-feeding rituals provides an excellent opportunity for parents to practice the gentle art of compromise and balance—to protect the toddler from harm as he or she pushes to separate, and yet to encourage the toddler to master the skills he or she needs to become independent. Fundamental to achieving this balance is an understanding and acceptance of the child's wish to master.

The Wish to Master The wish to master is right on schedule with toddlers, and it is an impulse that is essential all through life. Everybody needs to feel the desire to be able to do something on one's own—to say, "I can do it. Let me do it. Let me practice it." That is the feeling that makes the baby want to walk instead of crawl, get out of a diaper and use a toilet. It is the feeling that makes the child want to tie his or her shoelaces and learn to read. It makes the young adolescent want to meet new challenges in school, become skillful at sports, and babysit and find other ways to earn his or her own money.

Early on, this push for autonomy is the key characteristic of what is referred to as "the terrible twos"—a clash of wills relating to many behaviors, including those that relate to food. In some ways that wish to master can be very dangerous. The toddler wants to drink detergent, cross the street alone, jump from the bed after bouncing on it. These are dangerous, autonomous actions for which a parent must draw very sharp lines and follow very closely all the things that pediatricians advise—locking away poisons, keeping knives and razors out of reach, putting covers on electrical outlets and gates on stairs.

At the same time that protection is needed, *safe* autonomy cannot be squelched—practicing climbing in the playground when closely supervised; walking up and down steps, with you right there beside him or her holding a hand; playing independently; feeding him- or herself. In a high chair, the toddler is going to want to feed him- or herself and the parent is going to have to facilitate that by giving the appropriate foods in the appropriate amounts, cut up so that the child cannot choke on them. There's going to be a big mess; but the adult or parent in charge is just going to have to deal with it, put a bib on the baby and a drop cloth under the high chair, or wash the floor afterwards.

Feeding problems with a toddler are especially significant for two reasons. First, they happen at a time in the child's development when many psychological structures are nonexistent or just developing, and second, children at this young age do not have words to negotiate food issues. If you have a problem with a sixteen-year-old, that adolescent has a more established personality, defenses, and reserve; he or she has words to use for negotiating, and the ability to share feelings and to express him- or herself. One-year-olds, two-year-olds, and even three-year-old children cannot deal with the kind of verbal barrage that goes along with excessive control; lack of language compounds the issue far beyond "just eat the apple" or "just have your peas"—it adds an extra layer of frustration and the potential for a tantrum. This type of consistent pattern of control without language negotiation bespeaks a lack of empathy between parent and child that can't be dealt with because words are not yet available. Where a teenager or a school-age child can slow a parent down a bit by saying "You don't understand," the two-year-old cannot say that, and therefore the bombardment continues.

What Are the Risks and Benefits of Control? In sorting out what is safe and what is dangerous, this is the question parents must begin asking themselves of their toddler's desires. Obviously when it comes to running across the street, complete control is necessary for safety; but there are other areas, such as food and feeding, when rigid or excessive control may have little or no gain but rather a cost:

- Will it run counter to the normal development of autonomy—at age two and throughout childhood?
- Will it lead to tension that lowers the child's self-esteem and does harm to the parent-child relationship?
- Will it senselessly raise the child's anxiety about food?
- Will it work, or will it result in secret eating, gorging outside of the home, later eating problems?
- Whom is it really for—the parents' needs, the parents' guilt, or the well-being of the child? Is this control a feature of the parents' wish to live forever? Do they need to atone for being at work too much?

Thus excessive control can be an attempt to "make up" to the child real or imagined deficiencies in what the parents deem good parenting.

These are crucial questions, particularly when there is an impulse to exert control in areas that are not dangerous.

The Squirrels and the Elephants Relating control issues to "squirrels and elephants" is helpful in deciding what's worth making an issue about with a child—what is safe autonomy and what is dangerous—and what behaviors are really necessary to control. The parents have a big gun, but they only have a limited amount of ammunition. They've got to save that ammunition for the elephants, and not shoot the squirrels. So if a child tries to run across the street or put his or her finger into the light socket, that's something that warrants shooting off the gun. Those are dangerous, elephant-size issues. They involve serious, potentially life-threatening consequences, and they warrant a loud, fast, clear, and very firm reaction—a very large bang.

On the other hand, if you start using your elephant ammunition on every squirrel that runs around your house—every mess the child makes, every food the child eats—you're going to run out of ammunition when you really need it for life-and-death areas.

Practice letting the squirrels go by letting food issues go. In the context of the child's need for experimentation and independence, eating sugared cereal or an extra cookie at age two, or five, or ten is simply not a dangerous behavior—certainly not the equivalent of stepping out into traffic or drinking household poisons.

POSITIVE STRATEGIES FOR SELF-FEEDERS

- When the baby grabs for a spoon, give the baby one of his or her own while you continue with actual feeding.
- Don't worry if your child likes one or two vegetables, or

none at all. Fruits supply many of same nutrients as vegetables; offer those instead.

- Introduce new foods as "just a taste," accompanied by familiar foods. Keep offering them.
- Use a plastic drop cloth while your baby is practicing eating skills. With babies and toddlers, more food is going to end up on the floor or the wall than in the mouth, but self-feeding is still the goal.
- Allow for strong food preferences—choosing monotonous single foods, balking at others. Rather than withhold the favored food, offer a small portion with other foods.
- Try different textures. Shredded or grated vegetables are often preferred to vegetables that are served whole.
- Add pureed or shredded vegetables to sauces, soups, casseroles, meatloaf, etc.
- Encourage your child to participate in food preparation; the child will be more inclined to eat what he or she helped cook.
- Instead of asking the toddler: "What do you want for dinner?" ask, "Do you want this (name it) or this (name it) for dinner?" Give toddlers two choices, one a pretty sure winner, and give preschoolers three choices.
- If your child asks for more, give seconds.
- Offer the family food (chicken, spaghetti, etc.) to the child who only wants an egg (or whatever) every night for dinner. If that child says, "No! Egg, Mommy," give the child what he or she wants.
- Serve small portions and let children choose the amount of food they'll eat. If they don't eat much at one meal, their hunger mechanism will cue them to eat more at the next meal or at snack time.
- Have a ready standby or sure winner as one alternative. This does not have to be complicated or require a great deal of preparation—a simple peanut butter and jelly sandwich is always an available option.

From Child to Adolescent:
Rightful Teen Autonomy

In resolving issues of "safe autonomy," food and nutrition issues rank very low with adolescents. Teenagers are embarked on their own momentous journey into adulthood—a time of separation from parents in which the process of "letting go" is far more complicated for parents to resolve than it ever was with toddlers. As the adolescent approaches the adult world, the age differences between parent and child become highly visible. These differences create a natural, poignant tension. As one generation makes room for the next, the age-related limits of the middle-aged parent stand in vivid contrast to the endless possibilities opening up for the adolescent child. Understanding this tension, approaching it in a positive way that will serve the child's needs at this time, is critical.

Midlife Losses and Adolescent Potential: A Natural Conflict In middle age, usually for the first time in their lives, adults experience certain limits, or losses, in their life having to do with age. These may involve the realization that they cannot perform athletically as well as they used to, or that certain career goals have passed them by, or that a medical report indicates a risk of heart disease, or that a friend or parent has actually had a heart attack. Whatever the event, the middle-aged adult has no choice about recognizing these as facts; they just happen.

Handling this pivotal time—making the readjustment to losses that are uncontrollable and redefining goals for the second half of one's life—is a process referred to as the midlife crisis. While it is the rare adult who simply accepts the fact of his or her age-related losses without a struggle, most adults eventually stop mourning them by embracing the gains that also come with age, at the same time discovering new directions in which to go.

Some adults, however, never let their losses go. Unable to readjust to their midlife situation, they try even harder to control the people who are closest to them. They may become especially sensitive and vigilant to factors that may limit their child's future, act super-cautiously in areas that they would otherwise consider unimportant and that in their own child-hood they did not feel were important. The adult who resists losses will transpose his or her feelings about them onto whatever situation the child is involved in—be it eating certain foods or playing a sport in a certain way. That adult will overemphasize minor research findings, listen with a careful ear or look with an sharp eye for all the ways to control the child to compensate for lack of control over the losses in his or her own life involving longevity and full functioning.

This attempt at control can be even more intense in people who have had previous losses—for example, a divorce in their own childhood, a parent who died early on, or a chronic and limiting disease such as asthma. In that case, they will be even more rigid about trying to avoid the possibility of another loss in their life.

How does this perception of life compare with the child's? A three-year-old has no sense of his or her whole life; an eight- or nine-year-old certainly has no real sense of time in terms of a life span; an adolescent, if anything, feels at age thirteen or fourteen that anything is possible. An adolescent's potential is exploding in terms of athletics, sexuality, and intelligence.

You ask a teenage boy who likes to play basketball what he's going to be, and he will tell you he is going to be Larry Bird; that kind of drive helps him get onto the junior varsity team. You can talk to him day and night in terms of odds—that the odds of being as successful as Larry Bird are about one in 10 million—but he will not accept that. He will still go out there and think that there's a chance he can be that good. What motivates him to work out eight hours a day, come home late, stay up late doing homework, rush back into school the next day to take exams, and then play for his team is that hope of winning, of making it on his own. Luckily, trying to take that wonderful hope away from a young adolescent, and imposing the realism of midlife, is nearly impossible.

Because of their firm conviction—their passion—in everything they do, it is not easy to influence adolescents about their own mortality; in fact, for a parent it is impossible. Proof of this is in adolescent risk-taking behavior, not just experimenting with cigarettes, alcohol, or drugs, but also in their whole approach to things—the way they drive, the way they play football or soccer. A middle-aged person would never play soccer or football the way a fourteen-year-old does, for fear of getting hurt. However, as that fourteen-year-old dives to save a goal, dying is the furthest thing from his mind—he doesn't even *think* about it.

Teenagers with severe chronic illnesses may act as if the illness isn't there, and as if it makes no difference as to how well they function. The diabetic may refuse to take his or her insulin; the adolescent with cystic fibrosis may start limiting his or her physical therapy. A sixteen-year-old patient with severe ileitis (bowel disease) may absolutely refuse to take medication even though she's been through one operation and has enough disease again to require a second operation, which could be avoided if she'd take cortisone. However, she refuses to take it because it will to make her cheeks fat for a little while. She's a perfect example of how normal teenagers perceive a serious illness—as a defect in their body and in their future. Teenagers simply cannot tolerate any defect, any obstacle to their becoming autonomous adults.

Where a child at an earlier age might obey the parent's demands, however distasteful or unreasonable they may be, few thirteen- or fourteen-year-olds are going to listen to their middle-aged parents and agree with them. If a parent comes down too hard in support of any one issue, be it red meat or religion, the adolescent will take the opposite side. The adolescent is going to say "Get off my case" when cautioned about sex, drugs, driving, or what to eat. That difference, or clash, between the normal self-esteem, growth potential, and autonomy of an adolescent, and the midlife crisis of an adult, forces the adolescent to find his or her own way and allows the adolescent and the adult to separate. Otherwise, why would a normal, well-adjusted child want to leave the comforts of home to face the outside world, with all its difficulties, unless he or she gets some benefits? And among those benefits is a sense of autonomy, awakening sexuality, and an inner sense of feeling competent in making choices—including those involving food.

So telling a young adolescent to avoid french fries and pizza because he or she might avoid a heart attack at age sixty-five is probably the most unreal—and ineffective—way you could possibly pass that message along. It makes him or her want to separate from you and do the opposite of what you are saying. Minor quibbling certainly will have no impact whatsoever on the adolescent because the forces in his or her life to become autonomous are so strong that nothing you say will really matter.

As for health or food concerns, you have to be very sure of the nutritional information you're giving before you take a stand like that, and the odds are that even then it would take a tremendous effort—it will really have to be a priority of the family—in order to have it make any difference with a teenager. If you had a family in which cholesterol was a serious problem, for example, and you had a history of heart attacks at age thirty-five or forty-five going back for a couple of generations or across an uncle and a grandfather, then that qualifies as fair game for the elephant gun in that family—the family might need to make an all-out effort to monitor cholesterol levels and follow a low-fat, low-cholesterol diet. However, such a program would almost have to make that family's commitment as strong as in a diabetic family or a cystic fibrosis family—that is, high cholesterol would have to be recognized as a disease that everybody's committed to fighting, probably well before the child reached age twelve or thirteen. Even then, as shown by the resistance of seriously ill adolescents to medical intervention, you'd have a tough time monitoring the teenager's diet. Whatever the scenario, the concept is life and death, not what you eat.

Knowing that the adolescent's natural state of mind is to be stubborn or contrary does not stop some parents from trying to control their children, especially in families where rigidity and control is based on that very deep impulse to avoid loss, as described above. For these parents, food and nutrition (along with time and money) can become the levers they use to try to control their children in adolescence. And those levers will be held more tightly and more rigidly if that adult is in midlife crisis and facing those multiple losses.

Helping Adolescents Meet Their Body Goals One of the best ways parents can help bridge the generation gap is to show support for the adolescent in attaining his or her "body goals"—physical objectives that are all-important to adolescents at this time of life. An excellent way to approach this is by giving him or her knowledge on how food and nutrition can help achieve those goals.

Whether they want to be thin or bulky, for the majority of teenagers this is not a period of time when their goal is, or should be, to be as slim as possible or bulk up all the time. There are some exceptions to that—ballerinas, gymnasts, and wrestlers during wrestling season—but even then parents need to explain that adolescent growth depends on a good supply of nutritious food, and that cutting back on those foods to maintain a certain body weight or shape can, at this age, interfere with that growth.

It's a little bit dangerous to nitpick about food and eating habits; it's much easier to reinforce the adolescent's own goals: You want to be first on the track team? Let's look and see what you've done over the last month or two, and see how you can help that along.

In this respect, it is important to have a good sense of how well your youngster is functioning, academically and socially. If the adolescent is barely dragging out of bed in the morning, coming home with poor grades, falling asleep the minute he or she gets back from activities—these are warning signs, not only in the area of diet, but probably in other areas as well; these are signs and symptoms that parents can and should pick up on.

Adolescents, particularly those concerned about their physical growth, benefit from what is called a "growth velocity curve," which instead of recording the person's measurements each year, measures the amount of growth in a year—for example, four inches at age eleven; five more inches by age thirteen. Making a curve out of those points shows very quickly whether there has been good progress, and whether the youngster is going through a growth spurt on his or her accelerated curve.

TIPS FOR COMMUNICATING WITH TEENAGERS

- Make yourself available to them, available to listen.
- Do not assume they won't want to talk to you about their problems. Don't try to push them into talking with you but let them know you are there for them if they want to discuss anything with you.
- Share your concerns. Let them know what it is that worries you about certain situations or issues they're involved in. For example, if you think they are not meeting reasonable standards with their schoolwork and grades at the same time that they are missing meals, snacking on junk food, and staying up too late to get a good start in the morning, discuss your concern and explain why routines can help.
- Help them schedule their time if they are falling behind.
- Let them know (1) that eating well is the healthiest, strongest, and most attractive thing they can do for their body and their mind; (2) that choosing what to eat, and

eating sensibly and well, puts them in control of their life; (3) that food provides the energy that makes a person more attractive and better able to think clearly; (4) that dieting eventually makes it harder to lose weight (when the body thinks it is starving, it hoards fat); (5) that being hungry makes you think more about food and tempts you to "pig out"; and (6) that snacking on nutritious foods is great for getting calories needed for growth, at the same time doing away with hunger.

• Remember your own adolescence.

◆ ◆ ◆

Problem Situations

14

❖　❖　❖　❖

Problems
with Growth

Throughout this book, we have emphasized linear growth—
that is, upward progress as measured on the growth chart—
as the goal of nutrition in childhood. When a child is
growing within normal percentiles and thriving in all other
ways—is happy, active, and well adjusted; is developing
friendships and enjoying life—that's good evidence the child
is getting what he or she needs for good growth and development.

On the other hand, if a child fails to grow within his or her
usual percentiles as recorded at the annual visit to the doctor's
office (*usual percentiles* being defined as what's normal for that
individual child), or if there is no increase in length, these are
warning signs that, for any of various reasons, a problem with
growth may exist.

True Growth Failure

True growth failure can occur for a number of reasons.

Chronic or Recurrent Illnesses Illnesses such as bouts of ton-sillitis, one after another, or ear infections occurring every month can account for periods in a child's life where growth does not progress. Chronic infection of the ear, bladder, or upper urinary tract, intestinal illness, infectious mononucleo-sis or hepatitis in adolescents—all these can cause a decrease in appetite, inability to eat, or some other factor that, over a period of time, can affect growth.

Emotional Problems This is another area that may be an indi-rect cause of slow growth. Children who are grieving over the death of a parent or over a divorce, or who suffer from depres-sion, may lose their appetite and show a loss of interest in activities, have difficulty with sleep or school performance, and demonstrate a lowered self-esteem. They may lose weight over a period of time, depending on the intensity of their grieving or depression, but for the most part, this will not affect linear growth. Once the stressful situation is over, they go back very quickly to eating a regular diet and regaining weight. In any case, for any child who suddenly begins losing weight, the doctor will want to follow his or her progress carefully on the growth charts.

Parental Confusion over the Child's Diet Sometimes a parent thinks the baby or child is getting the food he or she needs to grow, and it turns out that this is not the case.

Six-year-old John was a good example of this. When he came in for an examination, he was the size of a three-year-old and his two-year-old sister was rapidly gaining on him. His mother described John's diet as consisting of about 3,000 to 4,000 calories a day, more than adequate for growth. On examination, John's digestion seemed to be normal: he did not appear to have any condition or symptoms of illness, such as cystic fibrosis, recurrent, unexplained fevers, or inflammation of the intestines that would make him need more calories than a normal child; yet clearly, something was not right.

Over the course of two or three months, it became apparent that for unexplainable reasons John's mother was overestimating his food intake. He was placed in the hospital for observation, and it soon became clear that in spite of the record of food the mother had kept in a diet diary, John's intake of calories was only 700 to 900 a day when it should have been up around 1,700 calories. The reason for this was that John's mother would consistently place food in front of him and remove it after fifteen or twenty minutes when he did not make any progress. She was recording what she put in front of him—not what he was actually eating.

Working with the pediatric "feeding team" in the hospital, John and his parents underwent extensive dietary and psychological counseling, and over the next eight months his intake of calories improved considerably. John began to grow and gain weight.

As in John's case, when a child who is not growing appears otherwise healthy on physical examination and has a normal medical history, very often the first step is taking a diet history and then "beefing up" caloric intake for three to four weeks to see if progress can be made. Once John's caloric needs were met, he began to grow normally.

Major Illness or Disease If a child does not gain weight with added calories or, more urgently, if he or she appears dehydrated or sick on first examination—for example, if there were signs of heart failure, or if the child were jaundiced or had diarrhea and blood in the stool—the doctor would obviously do a complete medical workup including tests to look for disease in the major organs. There could be heart problems from congenital heart disease, or hormone problems, perhaps a malfunctioning thyroid. Typical symptoms of thyroid problems are a heart rate that is very fast or very slow, skin that is dry, and behavior that is consistently very sluggish or else very hyperactive.

Most of the time there are other signs and symptoms of

these disorders *along with* growth failure that provide clues and help indicate which tests are necessary. For example, if a digestive problem were suspected, the doctor might do tests to determine if excess dietary fat were being lost in the stool, or if sugar was being retained in the intestine instead of being digested and absorbed into the bloodstream. The doctor might examine the child's sweat to see if there was any possibility that cystic fibrosis was causing maldigestion and poor growth.

It should be noted that out of all children, illnesses such as those mentioned only affect about 10 percent or fewer of all children. Also, with true growth failure, if the underlying cause is addressed, the chances of the child's catching up over a period of several years with no permanent deficit are excellent. Dwarfism or very, very short children pose special problems that are beyond the scope of this book.

Perceptual Problems with Growth

Sometimes a child is growing within normal percentiles but his or her growth or progress still causes concern. The approach to this kind of problem depends on whether the concern originates with the child or with the parent.

Concerns that Originate with the Child Children are usually not as concerned about their height as they are with being too short or not strong enough to "measure up" to their peers in various activities. Fortunately, most sports teams have a place for children in all varieties of physical size—for example, small children will play forward in soccer, bigger children will play fullback, and very agile children will be goalies. Puberty brings a new body awareness and, for most children, a normal awkwardness about their changing body.

Parents Can Help

Parents can work with their child to build self-esteem: most important, through showing affection, by setting reasonable expectations, and by congratulating or praising the child for meeting those expectations.

They can assist children in skill development by giving them opportunities to develop their particular skills, by helping them use their size to their advantage in sports, and by encouraging individual academic or artistic skills. (For short children, this can be a challenge in a society where tall people set the cultural standard, and yet role models who defy that standard exist in nearly every sport.)

For children who are disappointed about their height, parents should point out that:

- there is a range of heights among children and adults (there is no one ideal);
- there are similarities in height among family members;
- growth often continues through age eighteen or older and they may not have yet reached their full height.

Concerns that Originate with Parents In some cases, we see healthy youngsters whose growth is within normal percentiles but either because of some aspect of feeding or the child's appearance, parents think something is wrong. Often we see that common, normal problems related to food involve certain misperceptions parents have that can easily be cleared up. For example: (1) that spitting up is a problem and must be treated; (2) that young babies need food beyond a liquid diet; (3) that diarrhea is caused by diet and is always harmful to a child; (4) that an adolescent who becomes quite thin at the same time that he or she becomes taller is sick or should get more food.

Spitting Up A common situation in infancy that causes unnecessary concern is a baby's spitting up formula or breast milk during or right after being fed—in medical terms, gastro-esophageal reflux. This pattern of spitting up after a feeding affects about 60 to 65 percent of all babies, starting at about one to two months of age and lasting for about three or four months after that. Sometimes the baby loses less than an ounce of food, sometimes a whole feeding.

Spitting up per se should not be treated as a problem. If the baby is relatively content and gaining weight through this period (and most babies do beautifully whether or not they hold down food), there is nothing to worry about. With a small percentage of babies, problems with spitting up do occur. Occasionally they aspirate food into their lungs and that can cause pneumonia, in which case antibiotic therapy is required. Sometimes so much formula or breast milk is lost at each feeding that eventually the baby does not gain weight well. One common way of treating this is by thickening the formula with cereal—making it heavy enough so that it stays in the stomach and when the stomach starts to churn, the food does not stream up in the opposite direction. For the breast-fed baby, breast milk can be pumped in a bottle and cereal added, or feedings alternated between breast and pumped milk with cereal. If your baby is spitting up and not gaining weight appropriately discuss this with your pediatrician.

Fortunately, after about four to six months, most babies normally grow out of the reflux pattern and no longer need special attention—at that time, they're almost ready to begin with heavier, solid foods anyway.

If the baby is experiencing complications with reflux—for example, growth failure, recurrent pneumonias, or severe irritation of the lining of the esophagus, causing in extreme cases pain, bleeding, or anemia—the pediatrician will probably want to take an X ray of the upper gastrointestinal tract to be sure nothing is blocking the movement of food from the baby's stomach into the intestine, and perhaps do other tests that may help lead to a diagnosis of the problem.

Extra Food When It's Not Necessary When cereal is given to a baby who does not need it (i.e., who is growing along his or her curve), that baby can eventually end up very chubby. Usually that has no serious medical consequences, but rolls of fat are not necessarily going to help the baby, especially when it comes time to learn how to sit up and walk. The extra weight may delay these skills or slow them down. The recommendation for fat babies who get cereal too early usually is to give them more formula and less cereal so that they can resume their normal growth track.

Due to cultural pressure or other expectations (see below), it is often hard to convince some parents that extra food early on, or having a chubby baby, are not valid imperatives.

Toddler's Diarrhea Another condition that some parents perceive as a problem is toddler's diarrhea, also known as irritable bowel of childhood. The hallmark of this condition is a child who has frequent loose stools during the day. On some days the same child may have constipation, but in either case, the child will be *growing normally*.

The misperception is that diet in some way is responsible for the diarrhea and has to be readjusted, or that the diarrhea is going to be harmful to the child. We see children who have been through amazing diet manipulations to treat this diarrhea, either because the parent is convinced that one or two foods are causing it, or because he or she is determined to make it go away. However, as with spitting up, *children do grow out of toddler's diarrhea, and in most cases there is not much you can do about it until then,* unless the child is definitely known to be drinking an *excess* of fluids—i.e., two to three quarts of fluids per day. Decreasing that to about one to one-and-a-half quarts may improve or harden the consistency of the stool—at least in about 10 to 20 percent of cases observed.

Otherwise, if a child is happy and healthy and growing

along his or her percentile on the growth chart, there's not much else to do to eliminate the problem.

Diet Misperception in Adolescence The most common concern among parents of adolescents is actually connected with the normal physical changes that begin when a child goes into his or her teen growth spurt. Adolescents may typically start out somewhat pudgy and then, suddenly, within a few months' time, put inches on their frame and slim out. Observing these dramatic changes, parents can become worried that their pubertal youngster is sick, or becoming anorexic, or having a problem. The misperception is that because he or she looks thinner, the adolescent child needs more food.

In most cases, a closer assessment will show that the child is growing along his or her percentile and, if the child is functioning well in school and appears healthy, strong, and relatively happy, that there is nothing to worry about.

(If *any* child changes his or her weight by ten pounds or more within a few months up or down, then that's a reason to consult the physician and review the child's history and physical condition with the physician to see whether it is a normal pattern for a child at that age.)

Parent Expectations Parent expectations can cause unnecessary manipulations of a child's diet—and result in problems. These expectations, if they are apparent, should be sorted out and put to rest.

- *Is the problem concerned with accepting where the child is on the curve?* Some parents have a picture of where they *think* their child should be in terms of height or weight, and are disappointed by the reality. They may think their youngster is too short or slight in comparison with other children in the playground or school yard, or they may wish for a child whose appearance is an improvement on their own appearance. They may be disappointed that the child's size is not ideal for certain athletics or physical activities. They may worry that size will affect school achievement, thinking that a small body size means a small brain size, and a small brain size means less intelligence, when of course there is no correlation whatsoever between head size, brain size, and the scope of one's intelligence!

Whatever their expectations, these parents need to be reminded that in order for there to be a growth curve, someone has got to be at the top and someone at the bottom, and if theirs is the child at one extreme or the other, he or she is *still 100 percent normal.*

Also, that size has nothing to do with performance. There will always be small athletes who run circles around taller peers in the school yard or playground, just as there are whiz kids in math who are at the fifth percentile, height for age, and graceful gymnasts or ballet dancers who are at the ninetieth percentile, height for age.

Genetics play a key role, but sometimes there are surprises. Boys or girls in previous generations of a family may have been tall; the child standing before you may appear just the opposite. Thus the family stature is a helpful, but not a certain way of determining your child's ultimate height. In fact, there is no way to predict with 100 percent accuracy "ultimate" or adult height.

Usually, children will eventually fall somewhere between the height of their mother or father and if they have consistently grown along a particular percentile throughout childhood and adolescence, they will end up on that percentile for adult height. There are also ways of predicting adult height from X rays of the hand, wrist, and knee bones, but as with all estimates, occasionally there are surprises and the child turns out shorter or taller than the estimated prediction.

In any case, if a child appears to be well nourished and healthy and progressing along his or her curve, there is no need to be concerned about that child's growth.

- *Is the problem based on pressure to be "the good parent"?* Sometimes a child's appearance is seen as a reflection of competence—that parents are doing the right thing if their baby is chubby or, depending on the standards they hold to, if that baby is long and thin.

  Such standards are meaningless as it is difficult to predict where a baby will settle down on the growth curve during the first few months—and even during the first year of life.

- *Is the problem based on failed personal goals?* Some parents, because expectations for their own life goals have not been met, feel disappointment if their child is not perfect in every way, even if it means his or her living up to expectations that are unreasonable, such as size and appearance. Because they cannot control certain losses in their own life, they become more controlling over every aspect of their child's life, even including the child's growth. (See also "Midlife Losses and Adolescent Potential: A Natural Conflict," page 186.)

WHAT PARENTS CAN DO TO RELAX ABOUT GROWTH

- Check the child's progress on the growth chart and height chart (see page 271). Let the growth chart tell the story. If a child is within normal percentiles, let him or her alone to enjoy life's pleasures, including food.
- Do not make future predictions of the child's appearance based on what the child looks like now. As the child grows, size and shape will change.
- Talk to the child's pediatrician about your concerns. If you suspect your child is having a problem with food, do not attempt to diagnose it on your own or with a friend.
- Review the basic information in Chapters 8 and 9, which

may help resolve conflicts or concerns over growth or diet.

- Remember that a child's growth and development typically brings changes in attitude, behavior, and approach to meals and food. Adjust to, and accept, these changes by being flexible and by cultivating a sense of humor.

- Choose your battles and don't let food be one of them. Provide a wide variety of nutritious meals and snacks and let the child decide how much to eat.

- Set reasonable expectations. *Reasonable expectations* implies that a parent understand a child's capabilities and then provide the means for feeling successful in reaching them. In other words, parents should avoid expectations that doom the child to failure.

- Give the child opportunities. Without investing a million dollars in a sport or activity, at least provide the first step toward a chance to master or strengthen skills in an activity he or she wants to pursue.

15

♦ ♦ ♦ ♦

The Overweight Child

There are compelling reasons why parents should evaluate the situation carefully before trying to help a child with a "weight problem."

• *Intervention may be unnecessary, and it may even be harmful.* While the goal of overweight adults is to reduce pounds, in pediatrics the emphasis is on *weight maintenance,* not weight loss. In other words, a growing child who is five, ten, twenty, or even twenty-five pounds overweight is not encouraged to lose weight or to diet, but rather to *maintain his or her weight and grow into it.* That's a very different approach than weight reduction, which, by reducing calorie intake, also reduces the stores of fat and nutrients children need for growth.

Some children may eventually benefit from a weight-reduction program but only under close medical supervision and depending on their age (whether they have passed their adolescent growth spurt), on whether they are *extremely* obese (140 percent or more over their ideal weight for height, age, and sex), and on the length of time they have been fat (the longer a child is fat, the greater his or her chances of remaining fat).

For most children, a "watch and wait" approach is totally acceptable and in keeping with the goal of weight maintenance—*focusing on increasing physical activities, if need be, rather than on decreasing calories.*

In any case, no attempt to limit a child's diet should be undertaken without consulting the pediatrician or family doctor.

• *The overweight child is not always overfat.* Overweight means having more muscle that accounts for weight; overfat means more fat. However, most parents would be better off forgetting about the distinction as it relates to their child, and concentrate instead on that child's functioning, health, and happiness. While obesity can lead to chronic physical and mental problems in adults, being overweight may not cause a problem in children.

Obesity is commonly measured in one of two ways: (1) by determining the weight of the child and relating it to his or her length or height; or (2) more accurately, by using a skin-fold caliper to estimate the total percent of body fat based on the measurement taken on the underside of the child's upper arm.

Measurements obtained from either method can be plotted on charts and compared to national standards, based on the child's age and sex. By definition, children with either a triceps skin-fold measurement or a weight-for-height measurement that is 120 percent or more above the ideal weight for height are considered obese by current standards, and have an increased risk for associated health problems in adult years if they remain obese.

It is important to note that the role of early dietary patterns in promoting obesity later in childhood is surprisingly controversial, and most fat children do not in fact become fat adults.

There is controversy about the effect of being fat on self-image among children. Some studies show no differences among children, others show that children who are fat are very much the target of negative bias.

Fortunately, *most* children and adolescents who are mildly or moderately obese (and this is in effect an arbitrary definition) do not have serious physical or mental health problems as a direct consequence of their appearance or condition. Some boys may even be delighted in their large size, particularly if their goal is to be as big as possible.

• *The reported increase of obesity in children may be based on misinterpretation of statistics and measurements.* Although American children by some reports have become progressively fatter over the last fifteen to twenty-five years, there is conflicting evidence about whether American children *as a whole* have been getting heavier *in relation to their length,* which has also been increasing. One of the problems with quantifying fat and making correlations with length is that for research purposes, it requires a great deal of expertise and a lot of fancy equipment to make very accurate assessments. If the average height of the American child has really increased by a half inch or an inch, average weight percentages would have to be adjusted upwards, setting new, and higher weight standards.

• *A child or adolescent who is above optimum body weight does not put his or her health and future success in life at risk.* These fears are exaggerated among adults. Studies have shown that obesity in childhood does not correlate very well with obesity in adult years. One example of this, as reported in the *New England Journal of Medicine* (July 1, 1976), is Dr. Evan Charney's study, "Childhood Antecedents of Adult Obesity: Do Chubby Infants Become Obese Adults?"

With his colleagues, tracking 366 subjects into adulthood, Dr. Charney showed that while there is a definite trend for fat babies to be fat as adults (36 percent of the fat babies in the study became fat adults compared to 14 percent of thin babies who became fat adults), 64 percent of the fat babies did not end up as fat adults. In other words, a third of the obese infants in the study turned out to be obese adults, but two thirds of them did not.

These results were confirmed in a later study conducted in Denmark by Sorensen and Sonne-Holm, and reported in *The American Journal of Epidemiology* (Vol. 127, No. 1, 1988): Most obese children did not develop severe obesity in adulthood, and only a few had been severely obese throughout their childhood.

Why do some people end up with more body fat than others? Culture and environment play roles, but genetics provide the strongest correlation—*heredity alone has a 60 to 80 percent influence over how much body fat a person will have.* Thus, if one or both parents is slim, there is a 60 to 80 percent chance that child will end up slim, and if both parents weigh over two hundred and fifty pounds at age thirty, there's roughly a 60 to 80 percent chance that their offspring will be significantly overweight at age thirty.

This correlation has been proven consistently in twin adoption studies, where identical twins raised in different homes and by different parents demonstrate very similar weight-gain patterns, even though environments (diet composition, caloric intake, parental habits) had been distinctly different.

Energy efficiency, the rate at which a person stores fat and metabolizes it, is at the root of the genetics theory, but that has yet to be proven.

In any case, most children, especially adolescents, do not become overweight by "gorging on food," as many adults will believe, but by means of a number of other variables, including body makeup, that they may have no control over at certain stages of their life. Ultimately, the situation may change in their favor.

• *The health risks of being obese in childhood are very few.* While the top risks for fat adults are diabetes, hypertension, and joint disease, a child can be 20 percent overweight without risking any medical consequences. For example, a twelve-year-old boy five feet tall could weigh 120 pounds (rather than the average of 98 pounds) without any particular risk.

It is in the superobese group (160 percent above ideal body weight) where serious medical problems can occur and often do, and where even more serious psychological issues arise involving the impact of being fat on self-esteem, social feedback, peer relationships, sports, and development.

• *Weight intervention can lower self-esteem.* The superobese boy or girl forms our image of the obese youngster, but there is really only a very small percentage of children who are in the superobese category, and the rest of them should not be treated as such. Most of the children parents worry about are overweight by five to twenty-five pounds and are usually in the age range of eight to fourteen years old—a time when being chubby is well within normal. However, in middle-class families where achievement and appearance are so important to success, being even a little pudgy or overweight may be just as feared as being very overweight. That fear, relayed to the child in subtle or overt ways, is also overexaggerated.

Chunky, pudgy, or fat, no child should be made to feel bad about being overweight. A child's shape changes as he or she grows; excess weight may gradually disappear. There are periods during childhood and adolescence where children may be fatter or slimmer for their size, and then suddenly even out. You may see yourself in this—a pudgeball at twelve or thirteen who becomes pubertal at fourteen or fifteen, grows eight inches, and becomes a string bean.

Outlawing certain foods and snacks and criticizing food choices can lead to a no-win power struggle that sends a clear, negative message to the child that he or she has a "weight problem." As this in itself is more damaging than the presence of excess pounds (low self-esteem lingers on long after excess weight disappears), food and weight should never be made a big issue for children, regardless of what the charts show.

The child who is unhappy about his or her weight deserves support and attention to the problem; if the child is *not* unhappy about his or her weight and is within 20 percent of optimum weight, that child should be left alone.

Dos and Don'ts
for Helping the Overweight Child

- Do consider your own expectations. Do you expect too much from your child? Are you willing to change your own eating habits if they need changing? When it comes to food choices and nutrition, are you a good role model for your child?
- Do watch for signs that weight and appearance are affecting school performance or athletic ability, creating a poor body image, or putting limits on activities and social interaction.
- Do address the problem if the child brings it up; do not deny it exists or tell the child "You are fine." Share the child's dilemma; work with him or her to solve it. (See "A Step-by-Step Program for the Overweight Child," below.)
- Don't blame the child or the child's eating habits for a pudgy appearance.
- Don't suddenly focus on restricting or controlling food intake.
- Don't tell the child he or she will get fat by eating this or that.
- Don't obsess about your own weight and weight problems.
- Don't tell your child to watch what he or she eats or to go on a diet.
- Don't expect the child to eat one way while you eat another way.

A Step-by-Step Program for the Overweight Child

1. Check the growth chart, weight for height, to assess whether the child is truly obese.

2. If the child is within two or three major lines or curves (heavy curves on growth chart) on the growth chart, for example, 30 percent height and 75 percent weight—leave him or her alone. Depending on the child's age, it may be better to wait a few years and see if the child grows into his or her weight. An increase in height while weight remains stable would indicate this is taking place; if so, make sure the child has easy access to the foods he or she enjoys and observe eating habits over the course of a few months to see that the child is happy, healthy, and getting adequate food and nutrition.

Some children will remain as pudgy at age fifteen or sixteen as they were at ten or eleven; if this does not bother them, do nothing.

3. If there is a discrepancy of more than 2 or 3 heavy lines (see growth chart) for height and weight—for example, 50 percent for height and greater than 95 percent for weight—or if the child really thinks he or she needs to lose weight, then a doctor should determine that a weight-reduction program is feasible.

Very obese children, however, do warrant some form of intervention supervised by the pediatrician or family physician. Often we underestimate what it requires to deal with a very obese child, emotionally, genetically, or both. *Very* obese children are difficult to treat. Success comes slowly, athletic ability is limited, and genetics are often stacked against them, as is their social or cultural setting. We may dwell on the physical health consequences of obesity, but the social stigma for some very obese children can be debilitating. Some studies show that very obese children may do less well in school and do less well with their peers. The exception may be those who

THE OVERWEIGHT CHILD ◆ 213

find a special niche—the computer whiz, for example—but without a special skill, it is very hard for children who feel embarrassed about their size—especially teenagers—to overcome the ostracism of being fat.

4. Establish reasonable goals. Sit down and assess the child's activities and objectives—what he or she wants.

5. Take a five-day diet history, writing down amounts of all the foods that the child eats.

6. Make an appointment with the family physician or pediatrician to discuss the information gathered (diet history and goals) and what to do about it. If weight reduction is a feasible approach to making a change, work with the pediatrician to set a reasonable time frame. Once again, maintaining and "growing into" one's weight is the optimum for most children.

7. Establish a goal-reinforcing system tailored to the individual child. Use positive feedback for the child's accomplishments such as compliments on appearance, or giving extra money to buy a piece of sports equipment or clothing for the activity or sport the child enjoys—a new bathing suit, bike, hockey stick, tennis racket, etc. This will heighten the child's enjoyment of the activity, and will also encourage him or her to keep it up. Plan a surprise outing or trip together that focuses on fun, activity, and fitness. Openly discuss the positive benefits of the family's losing excess weight and keeping it down.

Special Considerations

Weight-Loss Programs Commercial programs that involve a timetable for weight loss and special foods are geared for adults, not adolescents. Adolescents need a longer time frame than adults to change their weight, and they have very different nutrient and caloric needs from what the system menu plans and foods can provide. It would be great if these programs developed the expertise and focused on very overweight teens; they have a lot of power and could certainly mount a very effective campaign to help teenagers lose excess weight. As it is, these programs should be avoided by teenagers because they do not take into account the needs of growing children.

Weight-Reduction Camps Weight-loss camps offer the overweight child or adolescent peer support in a comprehensive program involving good nutrition and behavior modification. Although expensive, they can provide very positive benefits, at least initially, in helping a child take off excess pounds, especially if the child is in the superobese category.

Regular camps, which are less expensive, are also beneficial to children who could stand to lose a few pounds as they encourage lots of physical activity. Children who attend, even for a few weeks, usually burn more calories than they consume in food, at the same time cutting down on idle snacking.

A Final Note

It takes time for a child to grow into his or her weight or burn off excess fat; as with adults, staying within one's optimum weight can be one of the most frustrating issues both for physicians and for the overweight child or adolescent. Eating habits are hard to change, and there is no convincing evidence that substituting foods really works, particularly when it involves favorite foods. The success of any weight program, as outlined above, depends on the active support, encouragement, and commitment of all family members. Even with all of this, however, the long-term (five-year-plus) results are very discouraging.

Our culture, with its emphasis on being "super thin," puts families and children under a great deal more pressure about their appearance than in the past. The extreme standard of thinness that prevails today has no known health or medical

benefits, but still it casts the idea of being moderately overweight, or even *normal* weight, as a problem. Thin, heavy, or
average in stature, *if a child is healthy,* then the notion of
acceptance by parents cannot be overemphasized or overen-
couraged.

16

◆　◆　◆　◆

The Thin or "Too Lean" Child

The thin or slight child—that is, the child with minimum body fat for his or her height—usually falls into the bottom range of percentiles for the child's age, weight for height.

There are good reasons to evaluate the situation carefully before helping a child who is deemed "underweight."

• *Length remains the most important aspect of growth and the primary goal of childhood nutrition, not size or weight.* Parents of thin children may worry that their child is "underweight"; they may try to coax or coerce that child into eating more food to gain weight and to put "more meat on his or her bones." From a medical and developmental standpoint, this is not a very useful approach either for the child or for the child's sense of well-being.

A child can stay as thin as a string bean—mean, wiry, and tough; tall and very thin; or short and very thin—and yet if the child stays on his or her growth curve for length, from a medical perspective, even if it were the fiftieth percentile for length and the tenth percentile for weight, the child would be considered healthy and fine.

• *Underweight is not necessarily undernourished. Underweight* can be described as minimal body fat for height (ballerina or marathon body conformation); *undernourished* can be described as minimal body fat and muscle mass and, as the condition continues, slowed bone growth. "Scrawny" or undernourished children may grow, but not to their full potential, as determined by their not following an established growth curve. On the other hand, thin children can be very well nourished, as confirmed by the fact that they are growing on their curve, doing well in school, developing socially, and enjoying themselves.

Tall or short, over a year's time all healthy children will increase in length. In adolescence, the increase can happen quite rapidly—at the peak of the growth spurt, even six to seven inches in a year. At other stages, growth is not quite so noticeable, proceeding in such small increments as compared with pounds that some parents need to be reassured that their thin child is growing normally. They can either check percentiles on a weight-for-age chart (see page 271) or pinch the back of their child's arm to see if there is some fat (keep in mind, however, that the young athlete may be all "muscle").

In any case, if the child is growing, leave him or her alone. Coaxing the thin child to eat more food makes no sense from a nutritional standpoint, and it conveys unwarranted concern about his or her appearance.

• *Heredity plays more of a role than food in determining a child's body type and size.* As stated earlier, genetics make a 60 to 80 percent contribution to one's habitus (body conformation), with culture and environmental factors making up the difference. Some children are genetically programmed to be stringy; some to have smaller bone structure, smaller chest sizes, and so forth. However, you cannot predict how they will end up because appearance can change dramatically. The slender boy may become the plump preadolescent who in turn becomes an average adult. Growth proceeds more rapidly in some children than in others—and yet it is very likely that a child's growth curve will eventually settle down to somewhere between the curve of his or her mother and father when they were children, and that the child will end up being somewhere between the mother's and father's height.

There will always be exceptions—the small boy whose mother was five feet, four inches tall and father was five feet, seven inches tall and who grew up to be six feet four. But even there, if you looked around at other members in the family, you would find an explanation. In this example, the boy's father was the shortest in his family, his mother was the shortest in her family, and there were a good number of six footers on both sides of the family. This boy's height, as well as the height of his siblings—a sister six feet tall, a brother five feet, eleven inches tall, and a sister about five feet, seven inches tall—sorts out just as geneticists would predict.

Age-Related Considerations

Infancy *Failure to thrive,* a term usually applied to infants, is strictly defined as the failure to grow in length or to gain in weight over a period of three months. This is due to a combination of decreased nutritional intake and/or certain problems involving the attachment between the baby and the parent. No one understands exactly the mechanism of what goes wrong, or how it affects growth, hunger, and feeding—but it does.

If a baby loses weight within a month's time or less—even if there is no obvious illness, diarrhea, or vomiting—that would warrant attention. Often the failure to thrive is a complex interactional problem involving an isolated mother, a family that's under significant tension, or a mother who herself had significant problems during her childhood between herself and her parents. As a result, the mother cannot adequately attach to that baby. Or the baby for unknown reasons may be irritable, hard to satisfy, or colicky—and therefore becomes difficult to attach to. Whatever the reasons, and without there being any blame, there is a poor fit between mother and child. What seems like a simple interaction—baby, mother, breast; baby, mother, bottle—then becomes a complicated matter resulting in a distance developing between the two rather than an attachment.

As those babies who do not gain weight over a period of three months are usually not getting enough nutrition, the pediatrician would usually focus on nutrition and nutritional intake rather than on heart disease, kidney disease, or liver disease and, at the least, would rule out inadequate nutrition before doing an elaborate workup.

Many people have a personal definition of the term *failure to thrive* based on their baby not looking as plump or chunky as their last baby, or not looking as robust or healthy as the baby next door or in magazines—therefore, they think their baby isn't thriving. Parents may base their assessment on criticism or comments from their family, when in fact the baby may be fine. Or they may have unresolved feelings of inadequacy as parents, regardless of whether it is their first baby or their second. They may think the baby is sick or, if breast-fed, not getting enough food. In fact, mothers who breast-feed their babies rarely have problems supplying enough milk. Nevertheless, that becomes the obvious concern when a baby frets during feeding, when instead the baby might be getting a cold or an earache or have a stomachache.

One of the nice things about babies is that because they grow so fast, you can very quickly tell whether everything is going fine. The baby in the first six months gains about a pound a month—the typical seven-pounder will triple its weight over a year. The growth curve shows progress every two to four weeks, and on those charts a pound for a baby really makes a difference.

If growth curves or a lactation specialist (see page 103)

cannot convince parents that their baby is on track, the pediatrician should be called on to observe how well the baby breast-feeds or takes a bottle, and to confirm that all is going well. In some cases if a baby is not gaining weight or appears not to be growing, the pediatrician may want to enrich the formula to provide more calories and other nutrients, as well as treat clinical nutritional deficiencies that are diagnosed—for example, give supplemental iron for iron-deficiency anemia.

If feeding is going fine and the baby is growing, then what is the mother really worried about? What is the problem? Sorting this issue out is a valuable exercise, especially where there is true failure to thrive, because these concerns are often more psychiatric than medical.

Attachment problems are complicated. Often they stem from the mother's own sense of neglect or abuse in childhood, leading to her inability to trust or get close to anyone. There may be tremendous anger about repeated rejection as a young child, a feeling that translates into the mother's feeling with her baby that she is being used without return. It is very hard to know how to give if you yourself were not given inner reserves.

In any case, the problem of a depressed mother and failure-to-thrive baby is a fundamental one that requires ongoing support—visiting nurses, health workers, therapy for the mother, etc.

The Thin School-Age Child and Adolescent If a child appears to have no difficulty keeping up with the activities he or she enjoys, no problem. Give easy access to calorie-dense food (see below) and stand back.

Dos and Don'ts for Helping the Thin or Underweight Child

- Do check for normal growth, especially with a thin or small baby.
- Do watch for signs that weight and appearance may be negatively affecting school performance or athletic ability, creating a poor body image, or putting limits on activities and social interactions.
- Do address the problem if a child is concerned he or she is thin, or if that child brings it up. Work together to solve it.
- Do consider your own expectations. What do you expect from your child? There may be no good reason for him or her to gain weight except in your mind.
- Don't focus on the child's food intake or emphasize weight gain by insisting he or she eat more or by coercing the child to eat.
- Don't treat the child as if he or she is too fragile—for example, by forbidding the child to play in sports or by giving the child the self-image that he or she is going to get hurt from being so thin.
- Don't make the child feel unattractive. Be cautious in situations, such as when buying clothes or interacting with other family members or friends, not to overdramatize a child's thinness or make that a point of observation or embarrassment.

A Step-by-Step Program for the Thin Child or Adolescent

1. Check the growth charts, weight for height. Leave the child alone if he or she is growing consistently along a percentile curve.

2. If there is more than a two- or three–major percentile fluctuation, or if the child is concerned about being "under-

weight" in appearance, work with him or her to achieve reasonable goals. Is it weight he or she wants to gain, or does the child have some other goal or body expectation that really is not reasonable—for example, to look like a body builder?

3. Take a diet history for five days and have it assessed by a nutritionist or physician.

4. Confirm with your family physician or pediatrician that your child's weight goals and expectations are reasonable. As with weight-loss programs, weight-gain programs for children of any age should be approved by your pediatrician. Children should know this.

5. To help a thin child get "back on track," keep meals and snacks on schedule and look for ways to increase protein, calories, and nutrient density within the basic food groups (see lists that follow).

How to Increase Protein, Calories, and Nutrients

MILK AND MILK PRODUCTS

- Serve whole or 2 percent milk, ice cream, cheese.
- Add powdered skim milk to regular whole milk (1 cup powdered milk to 1 quart whole milk).
- Use milk, half-and-half, evaporated milk, or sweetened condensed milk instead of water when cooking pudding, cocoa, milk shakes, cream soup, custard, eggnog, etc.
- Add powdered milk to yogurt, casseroles, bread, muffins, sauces, gravies.
- Add cheese to sandwiches, meats, potatoes, salads, vegetables, rice, pasta, and cream sauces.
- Serve cream cheese or cottage cheese on crackers; or add them to vegetables or pasta.
- Use plain or flavored yogurt as a topping for ice cream and in beverages such as shakes. Serve yogurt mixed with granola, or with whole-grain cookies.

PROTEIN GROUP

- Use fatter cuts of red meat, including rib-eye steak, hamburger, tuna packed in oil, dark-meat chicken with skin, dark-meat turkey.
- Add small pieces of cooked meat, fish, poultry, or eggs to salads, casseroles, soup, vegetables, omelets, noodles.
- Add eggs to French toast or pancake batter, custards, pudding, deviled sandwich spreads, cheesecake, or sponge cake.
- Use peanut butter with whole-grain bread; spread it on fruit or vegetables; blend it in milk drinks, ice cream, or yogurt.
- Add nuts to desserts, salads, ice cream, vegetables, or fruits.
- Add textured vegetable protein (for example, tofu) or cooked legumes (beans) to casseroles, soups, cheese or milk dishes.
- Include simple fried foods such as chicken or fish as part of the child's diet.
- Serve meat with extra gravy or sauce.

FRUITS AND VEGETABLES

- Blend vegetables and fruits with cheese or cream sauces.
- Add mashed fruit to milk, yogurt, shakes, ice cream, pudding.
- Make Jell-O using juice instead of water.
- Add slightly less water (¼ cup to ½ cup) when reconstituting frozen juices.
- Add honey or syrup to fruit in juice or vegetables.
- Add dried fruits to muffins, cookies, cereal, and grains or combine with vegetables, nuts, or grains.
- Add vegetables to soups, sauces, casseroles.
- Serve vegetables raw with a dip or cooked cream style.
- Add small amounts of butter, sour cream, or mayonnaise to vegetables.

GRAINS

- Make hot cereals with milk or juice instead of water.
- Use high-protein noodles and grains in casseroles and soups.
- Bread or flour meat before cooking.
- Offer whole-grain desserts such as cookies made with oatmeal, raisin bran, or peanut butter.
- Top muffins, toast, crackers, or pancakes with margarine, cream cheese, syrup, jam, peanut butter, cheese, or honey.
- Serve granola over ice cream, frozen yogurt, or fruit; or mix it with nuts or dried fruit.

17

❖ ❖ ❖ ❖

Eating Disorders

Eating disorders—emotional and interpersonal problems played out in destructive eating patterns—do not suddenly appear overnight or occur in otherwise normal teenagers who get into a fight with their parents and storm away from the dinner table. While of great public health concern, the two most prevalent subgroups, *anorexia nervosa,* obsessive dieting and severe weight loss leading to starvation, and *bulimia,* mild to marked weight fluctuations and secret bouts of binging followed by self-induced vomiting, fasting, or other forms of purging such as laxatives, occur in only about 2 to 4 percent of teen girls and young women and a far fewer number of boys.

However, as eating disorders are on the rise in a culture obsessed with staying thin, it is useful for parents, especially of adolescent girls, to become familiar with the characteristics of these food-related problems, which can have serious consequences: The morbidity and mortality rates of anorexia nervosa and bulimia are among the highest recorded for psychiatric disorders. With bulimia, the complications that result from the effects of binging and purging include diuretic-induced or laxative-induced hypokalemia (potassium deficiency); acute gastric dilatation, or rupture; and aspiration pneumonia. With anorexia, complications from starvation include diminished heart-muscle mass, dehydration, and electrolyte depletion leading to cardiac arrhythmias (irregular heartbeat patterns). Mortality associated with anorexia nervosa, excluding suicide, has been reported to be as high as 9 percent.

DSM-III Criteria for Diagnosing Anorexia Nervosa and Bulimia

ANOREXIA NERVOSA

1. Refusal to maintain normal body weight
2. Loss of more than 25 percent of original body weight
3. Disturbance of body image
4. Intense fear of becoming fat
5. No known medical illness leading to weight loss

BULIMIA

1. Recurrent episodes of binge eating
2. At least three of the following:
   a. Consumption of high-calorie, easily ingested foods during a binge
   b. Termination of binge by abdominal pain, sleep, or vomiting
   c. Inconspicuous eating during a binge
   d. Repeated attempts to lose weight
   e. Frequent weight fluctuations of more than 4.5 kg.
3. Awareness of abnormal eating pattern and fear of not being able to stop voluntarily
4. Depressed mood after binge
5. Not due to anorexia nervosa or any physical disorder

Anorexia Nervosa

The anorexic girl—and 90 percent or more of anorexics are girls or young women between ages twelve and thirty—develops an intense fear of becoming obese. Typically, she starts out overweight, or sees herself as overweight, and begins a moderate program to lose weight. Gradually the weight-reduction program escalates to drastic levels, either with severe restriction of caloric intake or severe restriction of food alternating with periods of binge eating and followed by self-induced vomiting or the use of laxatives and diuretics (bulimic anorexia nervosa). She continues to see herself as too fat—when she is too thin—a distortion that, by degree, can lead to a desire to become very dangerously thin. The intensity of the distortion in body image, and its effect on food intake, determines the seriousness of the problem and its treatment.

The classic case of anorexia nervosa is one with psychological highlights that may involve a pathologically controlling mother and her daughter (see below). However, there are other routes to anorexia involving social, cultural, mood-related, or biochemical factors, and these should also be recognized:

Athletics and Performance Goals With the rise of athleticism among young women in our society, athletes such as runners, gymnasts, and ballet dancers sometimes fall in a gray area called sports/anorexia, in which they starve themselves because they think being thin will improve their performance or, in some cases, because they are encouraged by their coach or teacher to become very thin. Many of them fall below the weight they need in order to menstruate. Many of them are in the bottom tenth percentile, weight for height, and still think they are too fat. Initial improvement in their athletic performance after losing weight reinforces their goal to keep losing, but eventually the weight loss works against them and may even motivate them to regain weight. This was the case with one very competitive runner who had gone so low in the athletic/anorexia mix that her running time had begun to deteriorate. The only way she would agree to gain weight was after her time improved with the addition of a few pounds. As with others who lose weight to improve their performance, her sports goals had to be satisfied before she would get back to maintaining an optimal weight for athletics.

Overvalue of the Cultural Norm of Thinness Well beyond the normal pressures most adolescents feel about being thin, some teenage girls and young women who become anorexic or bulimic do so because they are insecure about their acceptance by peers and see being thin as their best way to become accepted or popular. They may binge and purge to try to stay thin (bulimia) or they may never see themselves as acceptable and continue to go below their ideal body weight, progressing toward a state of starvation, to meet an unattainable goal (anorexia).

Another group of girls and young women cling to the ideal of thinness for security—for example, becoming anorexic or bulimic when undergoing transitions such as moving into puberty, or into high school, or into their freshman year in college.

Depression Depression is another element that can trigger eating disorders, especially when it accompanies transitions. With the adjustment to college, for example, about 20 percent of young freshmen women stop normal eating, perhaps doing so because they miss home and are depressed about the demands of life at college. That, combined with the social ideal of thinness, may merge to create an anorexialike syndrome, or a whole group of girls vomiting in a dorm, using weight loss as a way of adapting to or coping with their major transition.

As with the athlete, this type of situation does not meet the criteria of true anorexia nervosa (see below), as a full 20 percent of each freshman class does not end up seeing a psychiatrist or doctor for depression or excessive weight loss. Most of the women who get depressed somehow adjust to college, move on into normal activities with the rest of the class, and as their depression eases, maintain their optimum body weight. However, a subset of these women may have long-term personality problems and either because of depression, psychological makeup, or the way they were raised, lock into the more severe anorexia nervosa syndrome.

Biochemical Problems There is some evidence that there is a physiological base to anorexia—that young women who become anorexic may have some vulnerabilities in their brain chemistry systems that make them more prone than others to developing an eating disorder. They may have problems with serotonin, one of the brain chemicals that regulates mood and appetite. They may not feel hunger, or they may feel full faster, or when they are depressed, they may experience a change in serotonin levels that consequently affects their appetite system.

Correlations between faulty body chemistry and appetite are not far-fetched, especially when depression is involved. When people get depressed they change their sleep patterns, lose their sex drive, lose their energy levels, and may lose weight. One day they can work twelve hours; the next day, when they're depressed, they can't concentrate for fifteen minutes. Clearly, there is something biochemical that changes people's mood and hunger systems and may trigger what looks like an anorexia nervosa syndrome.

Psychological Problems Full blown anorexia nervosa involves psychological problems. Both in personality and life-style, the true anorexic is different from the normal teenager who is trying to lose weight to fit into a prom dress. The anorexic is a complicated individual who often has trouble with mood and interpersonal relationships, experiencing a certain amount of social isolation and low self-esteem. As young children, these traits may not be apparent; many anorexics are considered model children. They may be a little more intense than your average child; they may be a little more achievement oriented, perfectionistic, or obsessive, but most people could not predict that they're going to have a personality disorder, much less a specific personality disorder.

Some of them have very special relationships with their mother—a mother who is very different from the average mother, who worries about how much fat there is in the family diet, or frets about whether her child is wearing warm enough clothes outdoors in the winter. The mother of the classic anorexic may use her daughter to fulfill basic needs. From age one onward, or even as infants, the message the daughter receives relates to that need. Thus the mother-daughter relationship has a controlling quality to it, at least from the daughter's earliest perceptions.

Most mothers who are like this—and we have to emphasize again that it is a very low percentage of all mothers—will not be aware of the tightly controlled relationship they have established because it is so much an essential need of theirs, like breathing. Some daughters in this situation typically become secretive, inhibited, and private people, living in a kind of inner world safe from their mother's intrusiveness. Unknown to anyone but themselves, they may have secret food fetishes and food ideas even at an early age. In cases of true, severe disorders, children will eat very slowly or be especially picky as a form of rebellion. They will spit out food, hide food, or sneak food—very consistently. This is not just a normal tendency to occasionally sneak a cookie out of the cookie jar when no one is looking, or to chew unappealing food very slowly; it is behavior that openly or secretly conveys to their mother that she can control almost everything but she can't make them chew faster, or swallow. Food may be the last island of autonomy, and when these girls become adolescents, their cultural values, low self-esteem, and need for autonomy explode by

controlling food and losing weight. Initially this may satisfy
the parent and elicit a positive response, "You look great!" But
then it goes beyond that to basically telling the parent what
was intended all along: *You can't control me anymore because
only I can control what I put in my mouth.*

Even in this classic pattern, other factors such as a girl's
inborn personality, biochemical vulnerabilities, and the role of
siblings or father may all contribute.

Once again, it is important to recognize that only a very
small percentage of parents are intrinsically involved in the
psychological pattern of anorexia, and that simply being overcontrolling about food isn't going to create an anorexic child.
Most parents who are overcontrolling about food didn't need
their children to make their whole lives complete in a patho-
logical sense. They're just following all the advice that everybody's been telling them, or been selling to them about don't
do this, don't do that, and don't do this some more. They've
added a level of control because of the cultural mandate to
have good nutrition and because being thin is "in," but they
do not have a character need to be that way.

Boys and Anorexia As anorexic girls outnumber boys ten to
one, boys are not as well studied as girls, and yet the male
anorexics are often more disturbed than their female counter-
parts. In the college dorm you'll never find 10 or 20 percent
of all male freshmen vomiting to control weight—boys do
other stupid things. They drive fast, they drink, some of them
become moody. But they don't usually get into anorexia. So
the males who become anorexic are usually quite disturbed,
often having had very dysfunctional parent-child relationships
throughout their whole childhood, and there's a higher percentage of them who are truly psychotic.

With a boy who is losing weight and thinks he is overweight
despite being thin, a psychiatric referral is clearly indicated. In
other words, it would be better to skip over pediatric counsel-

ing or support and get a psychiatric evaluation right away because the odds that a serious problem exists are higher than with the typical girl.

Bulimia

Where the typical cases of anorexia involve young women who are often isolated and asexual, bulimic women are usually outgoing and capable of heterosexual relationships. Their food-related problem usually begins in late adolescence after various attempts at dieting have failed and they turn to self-induced vomiting, laxative use, or other means of purging such as excessive calorie-burning activity after eating to help control or maintain their weight. The bulimic pattern may be mild and infrequent—for example, rare binging and vomiting after moderate meals—or it may involve large amounts of food and frequent binge-and-purge episodes that interfere with work and social life. Weight may fluctuate but not to the dangerously low levels as seen in anorexia nervosa.

In either case, the bulimic is usually embarrassed by her situation, keeping it secret from family, friends, spouse, or physician. Following her bulimic episodes, she feels "out of control," guilty, shameful, and low in self-esteem. In time, she becomes so distressed by her symptoms that eventually she is willing to accept help.

Treatment of Eating Disorders

As soon as an eating disorder is diagnosed, vigorous treatment is recommended using every available resource, if need be, in an intensive effort to reverse life-threatening physical symptoms, regain physical health, and through psychotherapy, help eliminate the underlying causes of the problem so that the individual can increase self-esteem and proceed with personal and social development.

The variety of treatment options may include behavior

modification group therapy, cognitive therapy, long-term psychotherapy, and family interventions, as there are often family patterns that support the anorexic behavior. No parent ever wants his or her child to be anorexic or bulimic, but if that is the diagnosis, parents must recognize that they may be participating in ways that they may not be aware of to encourage the disorder.

David B. Herzog, M.D., one of our colleagues at Massachusetts General Hospital and a leading expert on eating disorders, recommends the following three-part treatment plan for eating disorders, as taken from the paper he co-published in the *New England Journal of Medicine* in 1985.

1. *Assessment.* In treating a patient with an eating disorder, the initial task of the clinician is to determine the patient's physical status and the risk of death. Indications for hospitalization may include (1) weight loss greater than 30 percent over three months; (2) severe metabolic disturbance; (3) severe depression or suicidal risk; (4) severe binging and purging (with risk of aspiration); (5) psychosis; or (6) family crisis.

2. *Education.* In the outpatient setting, the clinician needs to educate the patient about her disorder. A psychiatric consultation is indicated in all patients with eating disorders, to assist diagnosis and help plan treatment. The approach to outpatient treatment depends on the assessment and should be individualized.

3. *Therapy.* The severely ill patient should be treated by a team of clinicians including a psychiatrist and a general medical physician. As part of the initial treatment plan, an extended psychiatric evaluation should be performed, in which the patient can begin to experience psychotherapy and learn more about the disorder. The initial plan should also include behavioral treatment for restoration of weight or control of binging and purging, as well as ongoing medical monitoring.

INDIVIDUAL PSYCHOTHERAPY

Individual psychotherapy is the approach most commonly prescribed for outpatient treatment. Basic tenets for psychotherapy include acceptance of the eating disorder as an attempt to solve a psychological dilemma, establishment of trust through the therapist's acknowledgment of the patient's ongoing pain, and recognition of the multiple determinants of the disorder (social, psychopathologic, genetic, biologic, behavioral, and familial). The psychotherapist should avoid simplistic explanations or solutions. The therapist should also anticipate that some patients will terminate psychotherapy prematurely. Anorexics often retreat into denial when experiencing anxiety in therapy and may flee treatment early on. Bulimics may deal with their anxiety in therapy through increased binging and may also leave treatment prematurely. Antidepressant medication is useful at certain times, especially during depressive episodes and when the patient is ready to modify her eating behavior.

GROUP THERAPY

Group therapy should be considered as part of treatment. Group therapy is useful particularly for those who feel isolated by their symptoms. For the patient with a milder disorder, stable relationships, and adequate self-esteem, short-term dynamic psychotherapy or behavior therapy can be prescribed. Family therapy may be helpful if the patient is able to achieve only a limited degree of autonomy because of disturbed family relationships. For patients with a personality disorder, long-term individual psychotherapy is indicated.

Under ideal circumstances, an internist, nutritionist, individual or group therapist, psychopharmacologist, and family therapist may all be involved in the treatment of these disorders.

HOSPITALIZATION

While many true anorexics and bulimics respond to outpatient treatment, a subset of those will require inpatient treatment. Those who do are usually the adolescents who are so out of control with their disorder, or who have parents so unable to stop being intrusive, that the adolescents continue to starve themselves until they begin to have electrolyte problems—a very serious situation involving low body temperature, low pulse rate, low potassium, and problems with refeeding—a process that in itself is dangerous and potentially life-threatening if not handled by people who are experienced in doing this, psychiatrically and pediatrically.

In these extreme cases, hospitalization thus provides forced separation from parents (who may unconsciously disrupt treatment) and special care in the hands of those who know how to stabilize and refeed fluids and minerals to starving people.

Spotting a Typical Eating Pattern That May Lead to an Eating Disorder

If weight loss is out of control—that is, if a teenager loses sight of her original weight-loss goal and wants to keep on losing, that's a key warning sign of the anorexialike syndrome. A typical scenario follows, with our recommendations for handling it.

Sally, age thirteen, is making a concerted effort to lose weight. Pudgy as a preteen, she is making her food choices carefully and becoming slim and more attractive every day.

Over the course of the next few months, Sally's mother notices that Sally is becoming very, very careful about her diet and has increased her runs to six miles a day. In order to be reassured that Sally is not on the verge of anorexia nervosa, she can take these steps:

1. Separate out cultural wishes from a real disorder. In this case, all of Sally's goals—being athletic, being popular, being thin—are consistent with the culture.

2. Check height against weight. If Sally starts losing weight such that she is more than two or three heavy percentile curves below her height, that would be one clue, going back to the growth-chart principle, that she should probably be checked out with the pediatrician and the pediatrician should probably give Sally some specific advice about reasonable nutrition.

3. See if the pediatrician's advice works. If Sally stabilizes her weight and is happy being just a size ten, no lower, you're done. You've got a teenager who looks great. Reinforce that by telling her she looks great.

4. Watch to be sure Sally is in control. If Sally can't stop dieting, and . . .

- continues to lose weight even though the pediatrician has outlined some steps and has told her this is it, no more losing weight;
- feels that she's still fat when she's very thin;
- becomes more consistently moody, irritable, and depressed;
- cuts back her social relationships;
- spends every night alone in her room with the door closed, with earphones on her head;
- seems sullen; or
- demonstrates low self-esteem and a distorted body image, even though everyone is telling her she is thin

. . . all of this would be well worth a child psychiatry referral for the advice of an expert on what's really going on here.

With this sort of situation, you've got to begin to worry that she's out of control and can't respond to the normal cues. A number of things may be going on with her feelings. She may simply be experiencing mild depression and be having mild difficulty in adjusting to or overvaluing the cultural norm. She may have mild anorexia, and be needing to have autonomy and to sort out parent/child separation issues. More seriously, she may suffer from real full-blown anorexia with a longstanding personality pattern that's been developing since early childhood and would require major intervention. In fact there are a small number of Sallys who are truly disturbed who don't even fall into the severe form of anorexia and are psychotic and have very severe problems. There we're talking about one out of hundreds or thousands and this is a very rare way their disturbance manifests. There are actually some schizophrenics who will present and maintain an anorexia nervosa surface and underneath are truly psychotic.

Sally, and most girls and young women like her who become too thin, will respond to some reassurance and advice and will stabilize. The others will be out of control, and will need immediate medical and psychological attention, as discussed in the section above.

Helping Children Avoid Eating Disorders

- Recognize and accept what is normal: (1) That many preteens become plump as they enter puberty, and begin to thin out as adolescent growth accelerates; (2) That in addition to rapid growth, normal adolescent thinning can also result from increased athletic efforts, identification with people who are thin, and social pressures; (3) That the normal range of mood swings in adolescence can at times make food and eating less important to the individual, at the same time that her active, on-the-run life-style can result in normal decreases in food consumption; and (4) That the growth curves are dependable health indicators.

  Unless there were a major discrepancy with height, a

moderate five- or ten-percentile drop (i.e., weight on the fiftieth percentile going down to the twenty-fifth percentile) would not *immediately* indicate a serious problem. A *persistent* drop in weight is a clue that other issues besides food are worth considering: Is the adolescent depressed? Is she functioning well in other areas of her life? Does she demonstrate self-destructive behaviors? Does she think she is fat or have a distorted reality about her body image? Is she trying to hide food? Have you noticed her vomiting? Then you step up concern, look at the criteria for anorexia and bulimia (see page 226), and working with the pediatrician, evaluate whether the child's goals for her body are realistic. Children are at higher risk of developing an eating disorder if they start puberty early, have a competitive relationship with a sibling, or if there is a sense of limited acceptance by parents.

- If *any* warning signs exist, seek outside help, starting with the pediatrician or family doctor.
- Encourage the child's sense of autonomy and social life; encourage her to have her own values in terms of friendship.
- Avoid overregulating the routine aspects of her life; give her room to grow. Look for ways to give her responsibility for her own routines—when to get up and go to sleep; how to manage her rituals such as washing, dressing, and what to wear.
- Let her make her own choices about friends, clothes, sports, the food she eats, and how she wants to spend her free time. Involve her in the choice of camps, family vacations, and other pursuits.
- Do not become preoccupied with your own weight or convey dissatisfaction with your appearance. Your child will pick up on it.
- Help children through their developmental transitions. In words and actions, let them know you love them, are there for them, and believe in their capabilities. At the same

time, be aware of their special vulnerabilities (how they react in new situations), and whether they may be prone to depression during transitions.

- Prepare the college-bound child for being away. Line up friends for her in the area where she is going—peers and other adults. Visit her dorm and explore the area where she will be living. Give her a little extra money for treat foods or other items she enjoys at home. Send care packages. Give her an alternative to the college food—a hot plate, microwave, or refrigerator for her room.

18

❖ ❖ ❖ ❖

Food Allergies in Children

Allergies occur when the immune system, in a misguided effort to protect the body, reacts to the presence of certain foods or other foreign substances to cause uncomfortable or even potentially life-threatening symptoms—from mild reactions such as a runny nose or skin rash, to severe reactions including breathing problems.

The five most common foods known to cause food allergies in children are milk, soy, eggs, wheat, and peanuts. Other clearly identified foods include chicken, citrus, strawberries, chocolate, and shellfish—but *any* food can be on this list of potential allergens.

A Systematic Approach to Diagnosis and Treatment

If a food allergy in a child is suspected, it should be discussed with the child's pediatrician, who is better equipped than a parent to make a clear diagnosis.

To begin, the pediatrician will look at two areas—symptoms and susceptibility.

SIGNS AND SYMPTOMS OF FOOD ALLERGY

Skin:
- hives
- rashes, from blotchy red spots to dry scaly spots
- eczema

Respiratory:
- constant runny nose
- sneezing
- wheezing (asthma)
- cough

Gastrointestinal:
- frequent spitting up or vomiting
- frequent diarrhea
- abdominal pain/colic
- blood in the stool

SIGNS OF SUSCEPTIBILITY

- family history (when mother, father, or siblings have allergies, a child has more than a 50 percent chance of having them as well)
- symptoms intensifying after feeding
- symptoms persisting beyond other possible causes, for example, rash or diarrhea remaining beyond a viral infection
- symptoms in keeping with allergy (for example, a dry, scaly rash on the face and extremities)

OTHER CAUSES OF ALLERGYLIKE REACTIONS

Unless the reaction is rapid and severe—for example, an immediate case of hives or swelling in the face, or asthma or difficult breathing—it would be wrong to conclude immediately that a food allergy is the cause. Most reactions are not acute and can occur in children for any number of reasons other than allergies. These include:

Illness and Other Ailments Nearly all food allergies involve symptoms that are identical to the symptoms of common childhood illnesses—cold viruses, respiratory infections, bacterial infections, and in some cases, nothing more than a general irritability that, in itself, may have nothing to do with allergies and is not uncommon among infants, babies, and very young children.

A Temporary Lactose Intolerance Healthy, full-term infants usually have no trouble when fed human milk or infant formula based on cow's milk. However, during or immediately after a bout with diarrhea caused by an infection, some infants are temporarily unable to digest the lactose sugar found in milk. Once the infection is out of their system, they return to normal.

An Inability to Utilize One or More Specific Amino Acids in the Diet The most well-known of these congenital, metabolic disorders is phenylketonuria, or PKU disease, which is diagnosed by a simple blood test at birth that is now performed in newborn nurseries routinely throughout the United States.

Temporary Gastroesophageal Reflux This is frequent spitting up in otherwise healthy infants.

A Reaction Occurring Outside the Immune System A reaction to food could be chemical based rather than allergic, which can occur in some people in response to food additives or preservatives. Chemical-based reactions can also occur with substances such as monosodium glutamate, or MSG, the salty-tasting flavor enhancer that causes some people to sweat profusely, get headaches, or feel tightness in the chest. These symptoms have been referred to as "the Chinese restaurant syndrome" because MSG was once used extensively in Chinese food. While nobody truly understands why MSG causes this to happen to those who are susceptible (and actually it is a much smaller number of people than reported), the reaction in the body is chemical based rather than caused by an allergy.

Distaste or Aversion to Milk or Food Occasionally there are infants who do not like the smell or taste of the milk they are given, and they react by spitting it out or crying whenever it is offered.

Other intolerances include psychological aversion (negative associations), an inability to digest the food, or the presence of contaminants in the food. As a result of any one of these, the child may say "Yuck, I don't eat that food; I'm allergic to it"; the child may gag or spit up because he or she doesn't like the food or its smell (as with eggs); get a stomachache because of indigestion; have diarrhea because the food he or she has eaten was spoiled—all of which have nothing to do with having an allergy.

Parent Manipulation Children are fully capable of consciously or subconsciously manipulating their parents—such as throwing up right after they eat peas! That type of behavior can be replicated time after time, and it doesn't mean the child is allergic to peas.

Making a Diagnosis

A diagnosis of a food allergy is not always clear cut. Factors such as those mentioned above must be taken into account and, while the most effective treatment of a food allergy in a child is to eliminate from their diet the food that causes it, this decision depends on the significance of the food in the diet and, more important, on the severity of the allergic symptom in the child.

True milk allergy is probably only prevalent in about three out of one hundred babies—in other words, in far fewer infants than the higher numbers often quoted. However, because there is no form of allergy testing that can give a diagnosis of milk allergy with 100 percent certainty, when a physician sees an infant with what appear to be classical symptoms of milk allergy, he or she will often make the diagnosis without extensive testing. This is in the baby's best interest, as milk is the baby's primary source for nutrition and the first year is a crucial time when growth should not be compromised.

In most other cases, the following diagnostic sequence is standard procedure:

- *If symptoms are mild*—for example, mild spitting up or a mild-to-middling runny nose or cough—a wait-and-see approach without testing or eliminating the food may be reasonable for a week, as in that time the symptoms may disappear, indicating that allergy was not the problem at all. Certainly with mild symptoms, an involved series of tests or big medical workup would be too extreme— spitting up can come from a dozen or more reasons, and the runny nose might be from a cold.
- *If mild symptoms persist beyond a week,* the suspected food can be eliminated from the child's diet to see if things clear up and, a few weeks later, the food can be reintroduced to see if symptoms recur.

  Should mild symptoms recur, then a decision must be made whether to eliminate the food from the child's diet. If the reaction is known to be caused by an unusual food such as asparagus or mangoes, eliminating that food from the diet will not cause a major change in life-style. However, if the suspected food is found in almost everything a child eats—baked goods, desserts, pizza, snack foods—

and thus requires a major change in life-style to eliminate it from the child's diet, then the pediatrician should be consulted for advice, and more stringent testing should be used to be more certain that the allergy is "for real."

- *If symptoms relating to food allergy are severe,* that is, they make a child very uncomfortable, involve frequent diarrhea, rapid swelling around the eyes, asthma or difficulty breathing, then the pediatrician should be consulted immediately and the food that is suspected of causing the allergy, if known, removed from the child's diet.
- *In such cases, reintroduction of food can be risky and, without direct pediatric supervision, should be avoided.* If the food is not known, testing will probably be advised to confirm whether allergy is the cause of the problem.

Testing for Allergies

The need for careful testing is clearest only when the signs and symptoms of allergy are severe—for example, uncomfortable eczema, asthma, and other life-threatening allergic symptoms—or when the treatment must be carried out for a long period of time at significant cost, as in the rare occasions where a baby's or child's intestinal tract may be severely affected by allergic reactions to milk or other dietary allergens. In such cases, infants or children not only have vomiting or constant diarrhea as symptoms, but they also do not gain weight and, occasionally, will have blood in their stool. Testing—although not always 100 percent accurate—should be rigorous to determine if an allergic reaction to milk or another food is responsible for the symptoms.

Scratch Tests and Blood Tests In a pinprick or scratch test, a minute amount of some of the common dietary allergens such as milk, soy, eggs, wheat, or one of their components is scratched very superficially into the skin to see if a red, raised wheal develops over the scratch mark (as with the tuberculin test). In a blood test, a blood sample is taken and sent to a laboratory where common food allergens are mixed in to determine whether or not allergic antibodies are present.

The great value of both these tests is that when results are negative—i.e., showing that no allergic antibodies are present—there is a 90 percent likelihood that classic allergy is not responsible for the symptoms.

However, when the results are positive, the interpretation becomes more challenging because many people who show a reaction with a positive skin or blood test may have no reaction to that same allergen when it is ingested.

The positive test, therefore, only gives about a 30 to 50 percent probability that an allergen in question is the actual cause of an adverse reaction. Thus, despite sophisticated testing methods, in those children where the family history and the skin or blood tests suggest that allergy may be possible, physicians must also rely on "challenge and withdrawal" tests.

Challenge and Withdrawal Tests These must be done in a doctor's office under medical supervision, only after existing symptoms in the child have been cleared.

With smell and taste disguised, the allergy-suspected milk or food is introduced at twenty- or thirty-minute intervals in increasing quantities until symptoms occur or until the total quantity given is similar to what was being consumed when symptoms were previously noted.

This kind of "blind-placebo-controlled" test is best suited for confirmation of an allergy as the cause of adverse reactions. If no reactions occur during the observation period of three to four hours, the baby or child is sent home and observed carefully for signs or symptoms over the next two or three days, with a report made back to the doctor's office on observations.

The development of symptoms in a challenge test, together with a positive skin scratch test or blood test, is currently the best way to confirm if the infant is allergic to milk or other foods in the diet.

Food Substitutions for Children with Food Allergies

Whether or not food allergies are clearly diagnosed or merely suspected, it is important to tailor treatment to the severity of the symptom and not make more out of them with a child than is necessary.

Hypoallergenic Formula Those babies who have serious or severe reactions to cow's milk are usually switched over right away to a "hypoallergenic" formula with a protein component of casein or whey that has been extensively treated to make it less allergenic than the normal cow milk or soy protein found in standard formulas.

Soy Milk Some soy milks in the past have been labeled hypoallergenic but certain babies with milk allergies will react to soy just as they do to cow's milk. The advantage of the soy protein formulas is that they are cheaper than the truly hypoallergenic formulas and, at least for infants over a year of age, taste and smell better.

As there are infants who are not allergic to soy, a trial of soy protein formula may be recommended for infants who have not had serious reactions to cow milk. If there are no reactions to soy formula, then the infant can be maintained on the soy formula for three to six months or longer when a repeat trial on cow's milk can be carried out—starting in the pediatrician's office or hospital as with a challenge test.

Most of the time, children have an allergy to one specific food—for example, peanuts—which is not essential to their diet and can be easily eliminated without fuss or concern.

However, when the allergy is to a substance that is part of many foods—for example, wheat—then the parent needs to sit down with a nutritionist to plan a diet that meets requirements.

Reintroduction of Foods

It is very important to consider the quality of the allergic reaction in a child before reintroducing foods at a later date. If the reaction is severe, reintroduction can be dangerous. For example, if a youngster came in wheezing and gasping for breath after eating peanuts, the response would not be, "Gee, let's wait and see before taking the food out of the child's diet for a week, and then reintroduce it"—that might put the child at risk of a life-threatening reaction. (It happens that in the case of peanuts, children who show signs of a peanut allergy as early as toddler age will most likely have allergic reactions to peanuts throughout their lives.)

However, if a child has eaten a suspected food twenty-five times before the parents realized there was a food allergy, on the twenty-sixth time, with twenty-five previous mild reactions, the odds of a serious reaction with reintroduction are very low. If it only causes mild irritability, a slight rash, gas, stomachache, slight diarrhea, or headache, then it's fine to take it out and put it back in later.

Fortunately, many of the food allergies that are fairly common during the first two years of childhood disappear after that. While it is not entirely clear why this happens, it appears that over time the immune system becomes tolerant to certain dietary allergens. Milk allergies are a good example of this. Sixty to 70 percent of the babies who have adverse reactions to milk will have completely lost their sensitivity to it by the time they are two or three years old—in other words, cow's milk can be reintroduced into their diet with no ill effects.

In the meantime, milk and milk products must be eliminated entirely from the baby's diet, and a hypoallergenic formula substituted.

Among the 3 percent of infants who start out with a true milk allergy, a few of them will remain allergic to milk throughout their lifetime, and all food products that contain milk should then be avoided. As there are no hypoallergenic milks for older children and as calcium is needed to ensure good growth, calcium tablets are often prescribed for this very small percentage of children—although other foods in the diet, such as green, leafy vegetables, may in part replace some of the calcium normally acquired from milk or milk products.

Babies and Children in the Allergy-Prone Family

When an infant is born into a family that is known to be highly allergic, that is, where both mother and father have known allergies, there is about a 60 percent chance that the baby or the baby's siblings may become allergic to foods and other substances, including milk. The parents themselves may not be allergic to milk, but they will have passed along a greater-than-even chance of their baby having that tendency, or susceptibility. On the other hand, there is a 40 percent chance that allergic reactions *will not* occur in the baby—and often they don't.

So unless there were true or suspected symptoms of allergy in the baby (see page 241), that baby need not be put on a special formula immediately after birth. Breast-feeding is the first choice in feeding any newborn, as human milk is the least likely of any other milk to cause an allergic reaction. Standard infant formula is the second choice, but where allergies are present in a family, the pediatrician would be especially watchful for symptoms of allergy, keep them in mind when examining the baby, and probably overcall allergy if symptoms occur.

If allergic reactions to human milk develop or if the infant is not breast-fed because of parental choice, the pediatrician may recommend introducing a hypoallergenic formula in hopes of delaying the onset of allergic symptoms during the baby's first year of life. (Many of these babies, too, may be reintroduced successfully to a cow's-milk-based formula or cow's milk later on.)

With a second baby, breast-feeding once again is the first choice, as it would lower the risk of allergic symptoms. If not breast-feeding, then standard infant formula could be introduced with the guidance of the pediatrician to see whether signs or symptoms of allergy are going to occur. Milk allergies are not always present in the second child.

An infant in an allergy-prone family is at higher risk of developing allergy than an infant from a "nonallergic" family—maybe not to milk but to other allergens. Therefore, when introducing him or her to solid foods, your pediatrician may recommend holding off with certain foods known to cause allergy—eggs or wheat products, for example—until the child is one year of age.

Attention Disorders and Food Allergies

Are attention disorders the result of food allergies?

No way.

As outlined above, many different problems, digestive and otherwise, are mistakenly categorized as allergies—for example, chemical reactions to food additives, sneezing, or general irritability—but none of these can be considered a predominant or even minor cause of serious behavioral problems.

Out of the total number of children who have learning disorders, less than 1 percent of them may improve by taking a particular food out of their diet. However, diets that completely eliminate major groups of food for children or that put them on very restrictive diets—for example, the Feingold

Diet—benefit so few children that before being implemented, they require expert advice from a dietician/nutritionist.

No study has shown in any consistent way that a certain diet has either improved attention deficit disorders or other behavior problems. Teachers who have been with a child six or eight hours a day, in a classroom, cannot tell whether a child is on a diet, is not on a diet, has had a food eliminated, or has not had a food eliminated.

Given this inconclusiveness, food allergy is not a promising path to take for solving a child's attention disorder problems.

◆ ◆ ◆

Answers to Questions Parents Ask Most

Q: *My five-year-old seems to subsist on air and sugar. How do I make sure he gets what he needs to thrive and grow?*

A: First, track his growth on the growth charts. If he's on target on the charts and is otherwise active and happy, leave him alone. Given a choice of foods over a day or two, a normal five-year-old will pick out enough of what he needs, even though he only seems to be breathing air and eating sugar. (Parents who are still not satisfied can keep a diary of all foods for a week to see quantity and variety.)

Q: *Surely there must be some truths behind all the cautions about nutrition and foods. What foods should I worry about giving my kids?*

A: There isn't any single food that should be totally outlawed, but you should be cautious about consistently giving children foods that are high in saturated fats, for example, salami, coconut, or ice cream. However, this is a caution you should take for giving *any* single food all the time. You can go overboard on just about anything. For example, if you served lettuce exclusively as a vegetable at lunch and at dinner every night, that would be just as unbalanced in some ways as giving cashews (also high in saturated fat) for a snack all the time. Balance is the key, and cashews once in a while are fine.

Q: *When should I be concerned about the foods my child eats?*
A: If there is a really noticeable change on your child's growth chart, or if he or she is consistently making very narrow food choices.

When the youngster depends on very few foods for all of his or her nutritional needs, the risk of nutritional deficiencies increases. Early in life, infants depend entirely on a *single* food—milk—for all of their nutrient needs; thereafter, no single food is sufficient. With a two-year-old who only ate one thing and refused to eat anything else, you might have the pediatrician review that child's growth. However, if that one food were a peanut butter and jelly sandwich, with orange juice on the side, that would not be bad. On the other hand, if the child were only eating American cheese, or bananas, or celery, or applesauce, then clearly there would be a need for more of a variety of foods in his or her diet.

Ideally, the whole family should be eating a wide variety of leaner, low-fat foods—beyond that, we encourage parents to be reactive, rather than proactive, with children and their food. In other words, if a child is growing and developing nicely, we think it is better to assume that child is getting the right food rather than to overreact and try to change his or her diet. Children need to develop a sense about what is right and best; giving them food choices is an easy way to encourage this. If there's a problem—as indicated on the growth chart; or in normal school, social, and athletic activities; or in very bizarre eating patterns—there will usually be ample time to intervene.

Q: *My nine-year-old used to be a good eater but she has suddenly stopped eating the food I serve her. What do I do?*

A: Age is very important in evaluating a child's diet and eating patterns. At age nine, children are not growing very fast. Girls of nine are usually in their prepubertal period, and in about a year or so will begin to go into their growth spurt. A nine-year-old is most likely in the normal lull, and thus does not need to eat as much food. She may also simply be asserting herself, and that's more important, because nine-year-olds in the early phase of prepubertal growth are going to want to start thinking more autonomously. They may show signs of wanting to separate from their mother a bit, and decide on their own what they want to eat, and when. Parents should be ready to support this autonomy.

We'd be inclined to let this nine-year-old eat ad lib what she wanted, at the same time keeping an eye on her growth to be sure there were no extremes or a very narrow diet. The goal is to avoid a struggle about food, because sooner than later there will be plenty of other struggles that are much more important, such as those involving curfews, driving, sex, etc.

Q: *I know I should offer my kids a variety of foods, but it's such a waste! If they'll only eat cheeseburgers, why should I bother to prepare anything else?*
A: There are two parts to this question; one relates to development and the other to nutrition. The nutrition part of it is that fortunately, just like adults, children get hungry. If you don't put out the cheeseburger, they're going to eventually eat something else because they will get hungry, even if they are very stubborn. Remember, it can take repeated offerings of any new food before a child will accept it.

Remember, too, that children go through periods of monotonous food choices—and then switch to another round of monotonous choices after that. *Monotonous,* however, does not mean sole or exclusive food; it just means predominant. The predominant food stands out but if you watched them all day, or kept a food diary, you would see that they also had milk, juice, crackers, chocolate, tuna, peanut butter and jelly, or cereal, for example. Many parents only sit down to eat with their children once a day, which usually gives a very skewed view of the child's daily food intake.

It takes a little faith, experience, and the experience of others to know that children do eat a variety of foods although they do have strong food preferences.

Once again, if you are very, very worried, we suggest you and your child keep a careful record of what your child eats over four or five days and if there are more than nine or ten different items, relax—or review the diary with a nutritionist. We often do this when we are trying to figure out whether a youngster is getting an adequate diet or why that youngster may not be growing as we'd expect. A diet diary is one of the simplest, least expensive ways you can be reassured.

Give your children ready access to many different foods, recognize that they probably will not want to sample Brie or creamed broccoli, and if they have a cheeseburger for dinner and three or four other foods during the day, amen.

Q: *Do I put food out for my kids at dinner and tell them that's it? If they don't eat it, won't they starve?*
A: We do not recommend putting out just one thing for dinner and saying to a child, "Eat it or starve." That just creates unnecessary tension; it makes the food too important. It is better to give children a favored alternative, one that will not turn the kitchen into a cafeteria with six individual meals offered for each person.

In many camps and other settings where there are individual tastes, a choice is offered—either/or, with the "or" being something simple like peanut butter and jelly, American cheese, or some reasonable food that is an automatic, easy-to-prepare alternative. If they are old enough, the children can even prepare it themselves—make their own peanut butter and jelly sandwich—to share the work. Then, if dinner is fresh-caught fish, and the children do not like fish, instead of forcing them to "eat it or starve," let them have the sandwich and milk. That's nutritionally fine, it takes away the argument, and everybody enjoys dinner.

The parent has to recognize that everyone has food preferences, regardless of age. Parents certainly don't put out the same food for themselves to eat every night, especially foods they hate.

Q: Does the USDA food guide pyramid apply to children and, if so, how do I use it?
A: Inasmuch as the food pyramid emphasizes the "varied food message" it is clearly beneficial. However, the food pyramid has not made a major impact on childhood nutrition, and there is some concern among nutrition experts that the negative emphasis on the use of meat and dairy products will be taken to an extreme or misinterpreted by parents to think that these are foods that should be avoided.

In looking at the chart, the ideal is to try to increase fresh fruits and vegetables in the diet, and not necessarily to decrease the consumption of meat, poultry, and dairy products.

Q: What if they say they're still hungry after they've had a snack during the day, or before they go to bed?
A: Then they are absolutely normal! Let them eat all they want during the day. Try to encourage them to be active and follow their growth line.

Offer them a little box of cereal and orange juice, a glass of chocolate milk, a few M&M's, or a couple of peanuts—whatever they want, really. They have favorite snack foods. One advantage about having an adequate income is that you can have your cabinet stocked with food so your child can say, "I want this," and then go get it. That's a plus for snack foods, too, because your children don't have to depend on you to prepare them. Autonomy, autonomy, autonomy.

Q: *Television ads and peer pressure destroy all my efforts at instilling good eating habits in my children. What do I do?*
A: *Destroy* and *instill* are not words that we really agree with. *Destroy* is too strong a term for eating habits. You destroy a city, you don't destroy an eating habit. And *instilling* implies that you are going to do a transplant—of good eating habits.

There's no question that for a long time ads have influenced children to eat foods with a pretty narrow range of nutrients in them—sugared cereal, soda, candy, etc.

In fact there's nothing wrong with having sugar-coated cereal several times a week for breakfast, with milk or toast, or eating in a fast-food restaurant occasionally—the idea of outlawing everything that seems "taboo" strikes us as too extreme. (Interestingly, families in which everything is outlawed seem to produce children who are very aggressive about eating foods they shouldn't necessarily be that intense about. The intensity of their wish to eat candy equals the intensity of the mother's wish to destroy and instill the right habits. There's probably a direct correlation between the two.)

But back to the food itself . . . Even if children were to eat all the foods they are told to buy in the ads, they won't do so all the time and they are still going to end up with a variety of foods.

On another level, letting a child watch television ads provides an opportunity for a parent to sit down and talk about them, if you feel like doing that. There are ads for all kinds of things out there that you may not approve of for your child—sexy jeans, lingerie, violent television shows—but that they are going to find out about anyway. Giving your opinions in a reasonable way can only help the child learn to make informed decisions on his or her own.

Q: *Do I just give up the fight over healthy food? Sometimes I give in to foods that are bad for them but I feel so guilty about it.*
A: Give up fighting over what's healthy and what's not. The problem with taking that viewpoint is that it requires making

judgments about single foods and deciding whether they are "bad." Single foods should be put into the context of a whole day's food. Even if there are only five or six foods eaten by a child in a day, one "bad" one in there is not going to make any difference to the child's overall health.

Q: *How much control should I exert over when and what they eat?*
A: As little as possible. If you have a good reason, not a prejudice but hard data such as information derived from their growth curve, then you can maybe exert some control. Without a good reason, especially after infancy, don't do it.

Q: *If I let them have junk food now—high-fat, high-salt, high-sugar foods—am I setting the stage for health problems later on—high cholesterol, heart disease, hypertension, diabetes, obesity?*
A: No one has shown a link between childhood eating habits and disease later on. We cannot overemphasize that. Heart disease may have precursors earlier in life, but people's eating habits can change very dramatically, especially from how and what they ate in childhood. Any parent who sits down and compares what he or she ate as an adolescent with what he or she eats now will recognize that adults make very different food choices and have very different patterns of eating than in the past.

Diabetes does not occur by eating foods that have a lot of sugar; hypertension does not result from having salt on french fries. A child will not develop heart disease by eating saturated fat. An eating pattern that includes leaner, low-fat foods and continues over thirty or forty years may be able to slow the accumulation of fatty deposits in the blood vessels of some people—which is why the whole population ought to eat a diet that's a little bit leaner—for example, lean chopped meat for burgers, 1 percent or skim milk—but no single food even repeated in the diet is going to make a big difference.

Q: *Junk food and fast food—how bad is bad and what can my children have?*

A: As part of a varied diet, so-called junk food is fine, and "fast food" can provide quite a varied diet. Fortunately for consumers, the food industry has caught on to the idea that nutrition sells. If you look around the big fast-food restaurants, you will see they now have large nutrition charts in every outlet and nutrition information on their paper place mats. And children often buy more than just french fries these days; they buy a shake, fries, salad, and end up eating bread, catsup, lettuce, tomato, onion, meat, and other items.

Just because you can get your food quickly doesn't mean it is "junk" or "bad."

Q: *My neighbor's kids eat cornflakes for snacks and tuna fish sandwiches on whole wheat bread for lunch. I can see she looks down on the Cheetos and hot dogs we have around here. Should I feel guilty? Change to healthier foods?*

A: When you start to feel guilty, just think about that little ninety-year-old man who eats five eggs a day. Nobody has sorted out yet how much heredity contributes to long life and good health, and how much diet contributes.

A hot dog with mustard on a roll, a bag of chips or other snack food, and a can of soda or chocolate milk—that's not a "bad" lunch. It's a pretty high-fat lunch, and if the child were going to have hot dogs four times a day, six days a week, that might be a problem. However, a hot dog or pizza or tuna fish with mayonnaise once or twice a week is fine for a healthy, growing child.

Q: *Junk foods have all those "artificial ingredients" and chemicals—won't they do even more damage to a child's small body than they do to a grown-up?*

A: There's no evidence that so-called junk foods do any damage. And as far as preservatives go—to the best of our knowledge you are far better off eating a food that's preserved rather than a food that has spores and molds growing in it. The rate of illness would be awful. The same thing goes for the spray that is on vegetables and plants. If you wash your fruits and vegetables with water, there will be no problem. Water destroys chemical residues.

Some people have pointed out that there are more toxic chemicals being produced in your intestine on any given day by the bacteria in there that are fermenting on their way out of your body than in all the preservatives that are sprayed on or contained in foods.

Q: *I know sugar wreaks havoc with my child's ability to concentrate at school, but sugared cereal for breakfast is the only meal all day I can be sure he'll eat. Is this okay for him?*
A: Yes, it's okay. Sugar does not cause hyperactivity. It's hard to make an argument against sugar. It's a normal part of most foods. There's more sugar in an orange than in an average-size lollipop. Should you sit there and eat a bowl of spun sugar every day? Probably not, but if you go to the circus, cotton candy is fine.

Q: *My child is a skimpy eater who prefers snack foods to meals. How do I get her to eat breakfast, lunch, and dinner?*
A: Step back and ask, Does she have to eat breakfast, lunch, and dinner on a rigorously defined schedule?

A longer view of what your child is eating over the day is helpful, especially if any single feeding doesn't seem to satisfy one's idea of what the child should be eating. If the child eats an appropriate range of foods as snacks during the day—if a slice of pizza is considered a snack, or an apple, or a piece of cheese—over the whole day she may be eating breakfast, lunch, and dinner although not in the neat packages of time you envision.

It doesn't mean you have to cater to her every whim about when to eat food, or that mealtimes per se should be abolished; what it comes down to is the perceived difference between a snack and a meal. Children do not make that distinction all the time, often because when they are very hungry, all they want to do is satisfy their hunger. We usually think of a snack as a narrower range of foods—smaller number of foods eaten more quickly; not usually eaten with other people. But if you have two or three children coming home from school, they often all plunk down and have a snack together, and suddenly it looks like mealtime. The distinction fades a bit, especially when what they choose for snacks are "meal foods"—a slice of microwave pizza, a hamburger, a sandwich. For a child, really what's important is that he or she satisfies the hunger and gets enough to grow.

Should you worry about the child who comes home from school at four-thirty and has a peanut butter and jelly sandwich, and then two hours later sits down to the formal meal with the family and only wants a little bit of meat, a couple of french fries, and is done?

Certainly not. When you review the half a hamburger, the peanut butter and jelly sandwich, the milk, and the rest—from the time the child got home from school to the time the child went to bed—he or she really did eat an appropriate amount. All that child has done is violate the social norm of eating "what was on his or her plate," at the "main meal" with the family.

Q: *Some experts say that cow's milk may not be good for children. Is this something I should be concerned about?*
A: The problem with this position is that it is unnecessarily frightening to parents who worry that they will do harm if they continue to allow their child to have dairy products. There is no single perfect food, but cow's milk is a major source of a number of important nutrients for children over two years old.

Q: *Is whole milk bad for children?*
A: It's not bad, but over time it's not what you want. Looking

over the long term, with the goal of trying to lower the fat in all of our diets, there is no reason why the entire family cannot get together and have low-fat milk containing 1 percent or less fat. At a friend's house or a party, if there were chocolate milk or a sundae, that's not bad, as a single event.

There are also many children who are not big milk drinkers; they drink a half a glass of milk a day, or even one glass of milk a day. What they drink, as far as fat content, makes absolutely no difference.

Just as we wouldn't tell somebody that a child beyond infancy or an adolescent must have a quart of milk a day to meet all his or her calcium requirements, in the same way, you would be hard pressed to demand that a child must have low-fat milk whenever he or she drinks milk.

If the youngster were a heavy milk drinker—that is, had more than a couple of glasses a day—and if milk were something that the rest of the family drank as well, then you would want to go to 1 percent. And there is no reason why the whole family cannot drink the same milk.

Q: *My preteen daughter who has always been slender now suddenly looks pudgy. Should I worry that she is getting fat? What do I do?*
A: Wait. There's nothing more startling than a very slim preteen girl. Preteens ought to be a little pudgy because they're getting ready to go into puberty and they need the fat as a source for energy to support that growth. Body fat begins to redistribute, hips begin to widen; in other words, their shape becomes more grown-up.

We know one pudgy twelve-year-old girl who wanted a bikini and she and her mother fought tooth and nail about this bathing suit because the mother only believed in one-piece bathing suits. Why was that? the girl was asked; what was it her mother was worried about? "She's worried that I will attract some guy and sleep with him," was the daughter's reply.

And she added, "Yuck, *no way* would I have any guy touch me!"

Q: *My child and his friend would rather sit at home playing Nintendo and eating popcorn than run around outdoors. How do I encourage them to get outside and move around?*
A: Look at their activity level over the course of the day before increasing activity levels.

If a child has daily sports in school or after school, there is probably nothing wrong with coming home to play Nintendo.

If that child is in an after-school program, does that after-school program have activities? That child may be exhausted from playing an hour and a half of dodgeball in the after-school setting; he or she doesn't need to run around anymore.

Have a good reason for giving children access to organized activities—to get them ready so they can participate with peers, rather than fall behind the group.

Does the family exercise? Families come in complaining about the child being somewhat overweight, not listening, not getting out, and sitting in front of the TV all day. And then when one looks at the family, one sees three bowling balls. We ask the mother and father when was the last time they got exercise, and they typically say, "I can't do that. Too dangerous!" Interestingly, it is hard to get an adult to change his or her exercise pattern if that adult hasn't been in one.

The father was encouraged to take walks with his son, but he never "got around to doing it," even though he'd come in to complain of the child's not being active and being too passive. The child, in fact, either through genetics, modeling, or some other reason, was following the family pattern. If a child has parents who exercise, it's much more likely that child will exercise as well.

In the case of a thirteen-year-old, quite obese girl—a rock in front of the television—the parents had been just like her for the first ten years of their child's life, and just about the time their daughter was entering puberty, they decided to reform their lives. Call it a midlife crisis, but they both joined a health club, changed their diet, started to exercise, bought new clothes, lost weight, went to night classes, and stopped smoking and drinking.

Their daughter, who had been trained for ten years to be a slug, continued to be a slug. And there were vicious fights because the parents had gotten the religion of midlife reform, while the girl had stayed an adolescent. And in fact she verbalized her push for autonomy, saying to them, *I ain't running.* That was a difficult problem that required negotiation.

Activity can take many forms, both solitary and together with other people so that it builds social skills; exercise can take many forms too—from athletics to chores. (Raking leaves, for example, is a great chore, if you can get a child to do it!) The nine-year-old or ten-year-old probably does not need exercise in the sense of making his or her life longer. But that child does need exercise because of the social connections it helps to encourage—at least that's part of it. It also builds strength and positive associations with being physically active.

Q: *The statistics I read in the news show that children today are fatter and less fit than in the past. Should I worry that my child will be one of them?*
A: Your child is an individual, not a statistic. Follow cues given in your individual situation, not those dictated by population trends. Dire predictions and statistics need not concern you if, in your situation, they don't apply.

Q: *What's wrong with "playing it safe" and avoiding certain foods in my child's diet?*
A: That presumes you are categorizing foods, and for children there is no need to categorize foods into those that are safe

and those that are harmful. Many parents ask if "junk" food should be avoided. In our opinion, *only if it is totally replacing a child's regular diet.*

Q: *I'm not the only one in charge of my toddler's food. How do I know she is eating well?*
A: Check her progress on the growth charts.

♦   ♦   ♦   ♦

Resources

For up-to-date information about nutrition and other child-rearing issues, readers can contact these excellent sources:

> The American Academy of Pediatrics (Marketing Division)
> Northwest Point Boulevard
> Elk Grove Village, IL 60009

Write to request a list of flyers, brochures, and other materials available to the general public through the mail and at minimal cost.

> The National Center for Nutrition and Dietetics of the American Dietetic Association
> 216 West Jackson Boulevard
> Chicago, IL 60606-6995
> (Attention: Nutrition Info Center)

The National Center for Nutrition and Dietetics also has a Consumer Nutrition Hot Line Service (1-800-366-1655). Registered dietitians staffing the hot line can answer any food and nutrition questions, including those on food safety issues. Callers to the hot line may request brochures and fact sheets on specific topics of interest.

Your Child's Growth Charts

Find the child's age at the bottom or top of each chart. Draw a line straight up. Find the weight (height) along the sides and draw a line straight across. The point where they intersect is the percentile (determined by their relationship to the curved lines going from left to upper right on the chart).

GIRLS: Birth to 36 months
Physical Growth / NCHS Percentiles

GIRLS: Birth to 36 months
Physical Growth / NCHS Percentiles

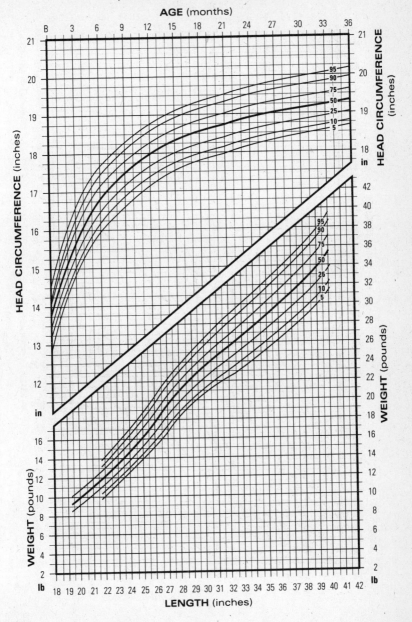

AGE (months)

HEAD CIRCUMFERENCE (inches)

HEAD CIRCUMFERENCE (inches)

WEIGHT (pounds)

WEIGHT (pounds)

LENGTH (inches)

GIRLS: 2 to 18 years
Physical Growth / NCHS Percentiles

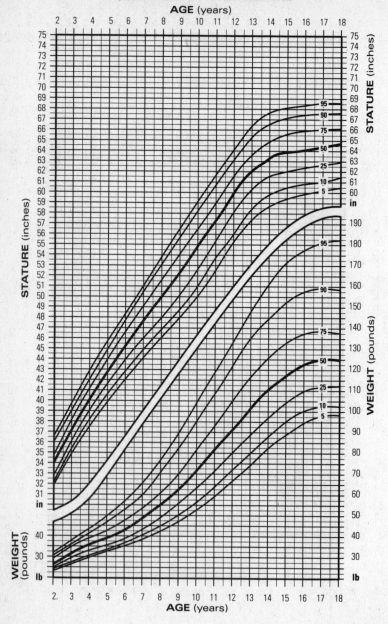

GIRLS: Prepubescent
Physical Growth / NCHS Percentiles

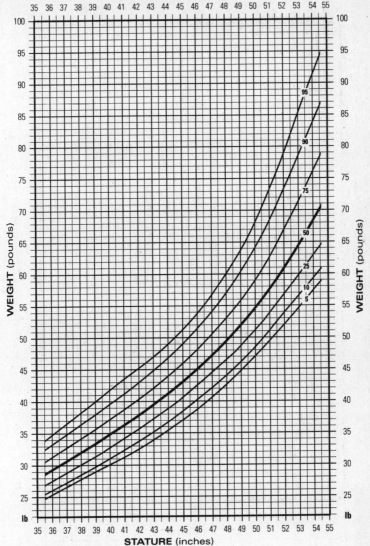

GIRLS: Birth to 18 years
Physical Growth / NCHS Percentiles

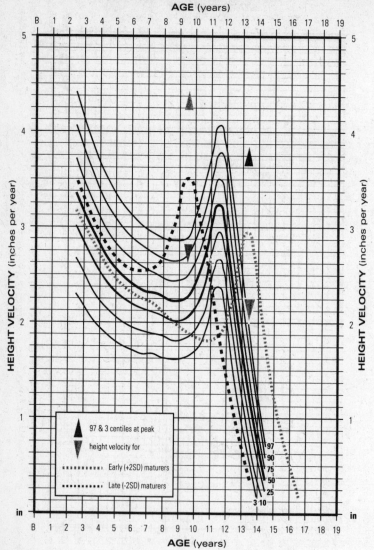

BOYS: Birth to 36 months
Physical Growth / NCHS Percentiles

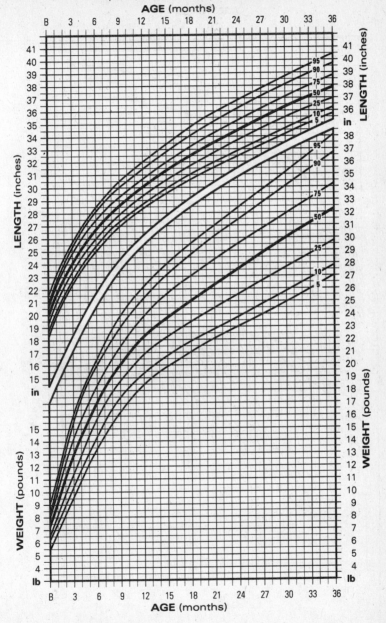

BOYS: Birth to 36 months
Physical Growth / NCHS Percentiles

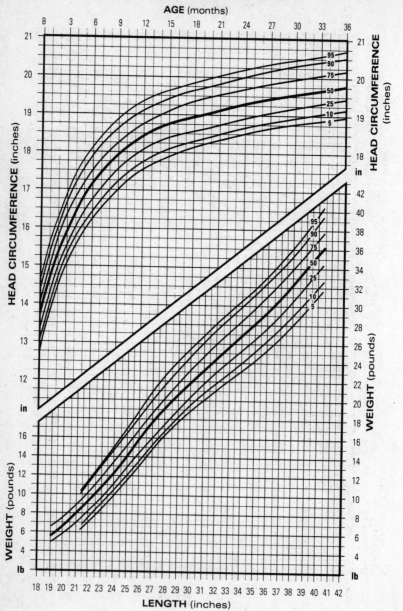

BOYS: 2 to 18 years
Physical Growth / NCHS Percentiles

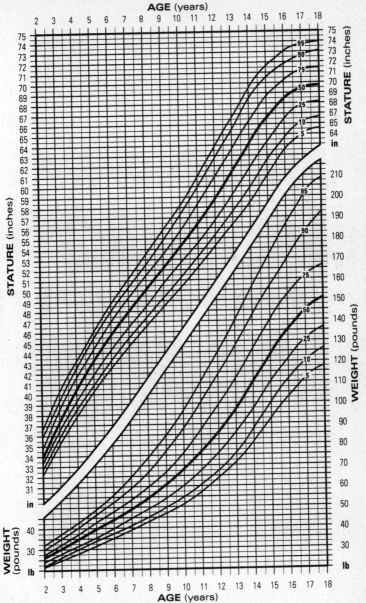

BOYS: Prepubescent
Physical Growth / NCHS Percentiles

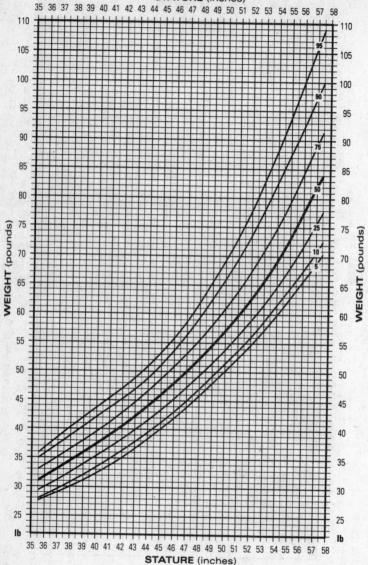

BOYS: Birth to 18 years
Physical Growth / NCHS Percentiles

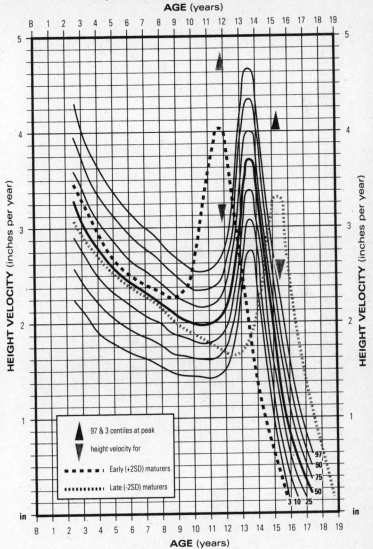

Index

acne, 171–72
acute gastric dilatation, 226
additives, food, 12, 19, 20–24, 46–47, 250; risks and benefits, 20–24; selling copy for, 70–71; types of, 21–24
adolescents, 9, 30, 50, 51, 60, 69, 183; body goals, 190–91; calorie intake, 95, 96, 110, 136, 138–40, 151; conflicts over food, 151, 159–62, 171–72, 186–92; dietary fat needs, 98–99; diet misperceptions, 202; eating disorders in, 225–39; growth and development in, 90–93, 95, 96, 97, 116–17, 138, 140, 190, 198, 199, 202, 237; low-fat menus for, 40; menu for teenage athlete, 139–40; middle-aged parents of, 186–90; mood swings, 92–93; overweight, 208, 210, 212, 213–14; physical fitness, 127, 132, 134–40, 266–67; risk-taking behavior, 188; self-esteem of, 189; tips for communicating with, 191–92; transition of child to, 186–92; underweight, 217, 220–22; vitamins and minerals for, 50, 51, 140; *see also* puberty
advertising, dietary, 64–77, 250
African-American children, 114–15
age of children, *see* adolescents; elementary school-age children; infants; preschoolers; toddlerhood
agility, 123

AIDS, 6
alcohol, 31, 188
allergies, food, 3, 20, 105–106, 176–77, 240–51; and attention disorders, 250–51; children in allergy-prone family, 249–50; diagnosis and treatment, 240–46; and food additives, 20–24, 71; food substitutions, 247–48; milk, 114–15, 176–77, 240, 244–50; reactions, 71, 176–77, 241–43; reintroduction of foods, 248–49; symptoms and causes, 241–46; testing for, 245–47; wheat, 240, 245, 250
"all natural," 72–74
American Academy of Pediatrics, 12, 32, 60, 66, 122, 165, 179, 269
American Cancer Society, 18
American Dietetic Association, 12, 18, 165, 269
American Heart Association, 66
American Journal of Epidemiology, The, 209
amino acids, 242
anemia, 107, 112, 200
anorexia nervosa, 202, 225–39; avoidance of, 237–39; diagnosis of, 226; sports, 227–28; spotting eating patterns in, 235–37; treatment of, 232–35
appetite, 11, 50, 117; loss of, 88, 89–90, 148, 196; natural, 11, 89, 136, 147, 154, 155

cheese, 36, 37, 41, 57, 75, 108–11, 114, 116, 119, 169, 170, 222, 223, 256, 258, 263
chemical reactions, 71, 242–43, 250
Chess (Stella) and Thomas (Alexander), *Temperament and Behavior Disorders in Children*, 175, 177–78
chewing gum, 168
chicken, *see* poultry
Child Development Laboratory, Urbana, Ill., 148
chocolate, 44, 65, 167–68, 171, 172, 259; allergy, 240
chocolate milk, 38, 57, 118, 136, 159, 160, 165, 170, 259, 262, 265
cholesterol, 3, 8, 29–41, 66, 68–70, 74, 98, 99, 110, 112, 153, 189, 261; in children, testing for, 32–35, 74; dietary guidelines and applications, 36–41; function of, 29–30; LDL factor, 31–32, 34–35
"cholesterol-free," 74
chromium, 54
chronic illnesses, 196
cigarettes, 31, 34, 188
citrates, 71
coaches, 125, 142, 227
coconuts, 30, 36, 72, 167, 255
cognitive therapy, 233
cold cuts, 21, 24, 27, 160
cold foods, 25, 27
cold viruses, 242
colic, 174, 176–77, 219, 241
college, 228–29, 239
colon cancer, 57, 112, 120
color additives, 21, 24, 70–71
colostrum, 101
combination drinks, 119
competitive sports, 126–27, 141
concentrating juices, 75
conflict-free meals, hints for, 154–56
conflicts, food, 145–92; food tensions at transition stages, 173–92; "junk food" dilemma, 164–72; mealtime difficulties, 147–63; parental overcontrol of food, 4–8, 93–94, 148, 159–60, 170–72, 176, 181–92, 199, 202–11, 230–31, 255–68
constipation, 56, 201
contamination, food, 18, 21, 23–28
cookies, 44, 111, 118, 119, 160, 161, 224
coordination, 124
copper, 54, 111
corn oil, 30, 36, 41
cornstarch, 75
corn syrup, 20, 44
cow's milk, 100, 107, 108, 177, 242, 247, 248, 250, 264

crackers, 118, 121, 161, 222
cramps, 115
cream, 36, 41
Cream of Wheat, 114
crying infants, 173–81
cultural factors, in growth and development, 93, 94, 209, 217, 228
cutting boards, 25, 27
cystic fibrosis, 188, 189, 196, 198

dairy products, 98, 259, 264; allergy, 114–15, 176–77, 240, 244, 245, 248–49; in child's diet, 99–104, 106, 108–14, 116, 118, 121; low-fat, 37, 38, 41, 108–14, 154, 159, 261, 265; for underweight child, 222; *see also specific foods*
Davis, Clara, 152
day care, 102
death, 9, 187, 196, 225, 226
dehydration, 226
Delaney, Clause, 20
Denmark, 209
depression, and eating disorders, 228–29, 233, 234, 236, 238
deprivation, desire heightened by, 12
desserts, 156, 244; low-fat, 41
diabetes, 5, 44, 188, 189, 209, 261
diarrhea, 45, 73, 74, 115, 177, 196, 199, 218; and allergies, 241–44, 248; toddler's, 201–202
diary, food, 257–58
diet, 95–121; calorie intake, 95–97, 104, 110, 113, 116, 148–52, 196–97, 206; for children, 105, 108–21; for energy, 95–98; erratic eating, 10–11, 148–54; fat in, 98–99; favorite food choices, 110–11; for growth and development, 95–121; for infants, 99–108, 117; mealtime difficulties, 147–63; monotonous, 152–53, 256–57; parental confusion over, 196–97; parental overcontrol of, 4–8, 93–94, 148, 159–60, 170–72, 176, 181–92, 199, 202–11, 230–31, 255–68; perceptual problems with, 198–204; recommended dietary allowances, 109–10; snacks in, 116–19; and sports, 50–54, 135–40; transition to solid foods, 104–108, 152, varied, 108–10, 152, 153, 256–58; vegetarian, 51, 121; vitamins and minerals in, 106–16, 119, 120, 121; *see also* growth and development; *specific age groups and foods*
diet soda, 168–69
digestion, 29, 179–80; and fiber, 55–58; problems, 196–200, 241, 243, 245

diet, 106–12, 116, 119–21; fiber,
55–58; pesticides used on, 18–19, 74,
120, 263; sugar in, 44; for underweight
child, 223
fruit juices, 6, 44, 45, 54, 73, 75, 106,
113, 115, 118, 136, 158, 159, 160,
162, 223, 224, 256; from concentrate,
75; as snack, 118, 119

gallstones, 36
games, food, 8
gelatin, 24
genetics, 10, 30, 31, 68, 69, 84, 115, 140,
241, 266; and growth patterns, 84, 86,
93, 203, 217; and obesity, 209, 212;
and underweight, 217–18
girls, 116, 257; adolescent growth,
90–93, 110, 116–17, 138, 140, 225,
266–67; calorie intake, 110, 116–17,
138; eating disorders in, 225–39;
hyperactive, 46; preteen, 265–66; see
also specific age groups
good eating habits, 9–10
goodness of fit, in mother-baby
relationship, 175–76
grains, 37, 98; in child's diet, 106–14,
116, 121; fiber, 55–58; for
underweight child, 224
grandparents, and junk food conflicts,
165–66, 171
granola, 72
grapes, 108, 161
GRAS list (Generally Recognized As
Safe), 20
grasp-and-release skills, 127
Greece, 69
group therapy, 234
growth and development, 8, 9, 10, 12,
29, 37, 81–94, 124, 156; in
adolescence, 90–93, 95, 96, 97,
116–17, 138, 140, 190, 198, 199, 202,
237; age two to age ten, 89–90, 93,
96, 98, 153; calorie intake, 9–97, 104,
110, 113, 116, 148–52, 196–97, 206;
cholesterol and fat in, 29–30, 36–38,
98–99; diet for, 95–121; energy
connection, 95–97; genetic factors, 84,
86, 93, 203, 217; growth curves, 83,
88, 156, 191, 195, 202–204, 212,
216–19, 237; growth failure, 195–98;
in infancy, 82–89, 93, 96, 97, 98,
99–104, 219; long-term view of,
81–94; perceptual problems with,
198–204; and physical fitness, 122–43;
problems with, 195–205; vitamins and
minerals in, 48–54, 106–16; see also
diet; height; specific age groups and
foods; weight

growth failure, 195–98
growth velocity curve, 191
guar gum, 70
guilt, 4, 6, 166, 175, 183, 232, 260, 262
gymnastics, 130

Halloween, 171
hamburgers, 257, 264
handling food, 24–28
Harvard School of Public Health, 91
health-related fitness, 123
heart, 30, 123
heart arrhythmia, 52, 226
heart disease, 9, 52, 55, 64, 68, 69, 153,
186, 189, 197, 219, 226, 261; role of
cholesterol and fat in, 30–35, 66,
69–70
height, 81, 83, 203, 216; and genetics,
209, 212, 217–18; growth failure,
195–98; perceptual problems with,
198–205; in stages of growth, 81–94,
110; -for-weight measurement, 207,
208, 210, 212, 216–17, 221, 236–38,
271; see also growth and development
hematocrit, 51, 112
hepatitis, 196
herbal tea, 119
heredity, 10, 34, 68, 69, 209, 217, 241,
262; see also genetics
Herzog, David B., 91, 233
high blood pressure, 34, 67–68, 76, 209,
261
high chair, 105, 181, 182
high-density lipoproteins (HDL), 31
high-energy foods, 97–98
hives, 241
home-canned foods, 18–19
home food safety, 24–28
homework, 61, 163, 187, 191
honey, 18, 44, 73, 223
hormones, 35, 45, 52, 115; imbalances,
87, 197; and menstruation, 91–92
hospitalization, for eating disorders, 235
hot dogs, 108, 165, 262
hot foods, 25, 28
hyperactivity, 12, 21, 112, 197; and
sugar, 42–43, 46–47, 62, 263
hypoallergenic formula, 247, 249, 250
hypokalemia, 226

ice cream, 14, 20, 28, 41, 110, 111, 154,
222, 223, 224, 225
ice skating, 130
IGF-1, 22
ileitis, 188
illness, 218, 242; chronic, 196; major,
197–98; see also specific illnesses

About the Authors

A practicing pediatrician for the past twenty years, RONALD R. KLEIN-
MAN, M.D., is chief of the division of Pediatric Gastroenterology and
Nutrition at Massachusetts General Hospital. He is also associate
professor of pediatrics at Harvard Medical School and former chair-
man of the Committee on Nutrition of the American Academy of
Pediatrics. MICHAEL S. JELLINEK, M.D., is chief of the Child Psychiatry
Service at Massachusetts General Hospital, and associate professor
of psychiatry (pediatrics) at Harvard Medical School. JULIE HOUSTON
has worked in book publishing for the past thirty years as an editor
and a freelance writer. She has co-authored five books on health and
family, and her writing has appeared in *Parents* magazine. She lives
in Brooklyn.